MOSBY'S 1998
ASSESSTEST

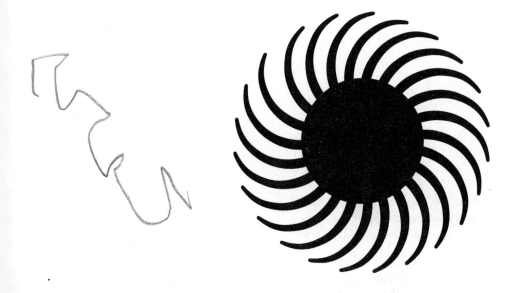

A practice exam for RN licensure

SAXTON ♦ PELIKAN ♦ GREEN

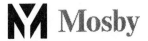 Mosby

St. Louis Baltimore Boston Carlsbad Chicago Minneapolis New York Philadelphia Portland
London Milan Sydney Tokyo Toronto

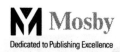
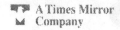

Mosby

Dedicated to Publishing Excellence

A Times Mirror
Company

Publisher: Nancy L. Coon
Editor: Loren S. Wilson
Developmental Editor: Glenn Floyd
Manufacturing Supervisor: Don Carlisle

Printed in the United States of America
Composition by Mosby Electronic Publishing
Printing/binding by Plus Communications

Mosby, Inc.
11830 Westline Industrial Drive
St. Louis, Missouri 63146

International Standard Book Number 0-8151-8508-1

97 98 99 00 01 / 9 8 7 6 5 4 3 2 1

Editorial Panel

Carol Flaugher, R.N., B.S.N., M.S.

State University of New York at Buffalo School of
    Nursing
Buffalo, New York

Doris E. Nicholas, R.N., B.S., M.S., Ph.D.

Howard University College of Nursing
Washington, District of Columbia

Anita Throwe, R.N., B.S.N., M.S.

Medical University of South Carolina, College of
    Nursing
Florence, South Carolina

Janet T. Ihlenfeld, R.N., B.S.N., M.S.N., Ph.D.

D'Youville College
Buffalo, New York

Carole J. Labby, R.N., B.S.N., M.S.

College of the Mainland
Houston, Texas

Mary Reuther Herring, R.N., B.S.N., M.S.N.

Motorola Incorporated and University of Phoenix
Phoenix, Arizonia

Pamela M. Lemmon, R.N., B.S.N., M.S.N.

Gannon University
Youngstown, Ohio

Ellen M. Chiocca, R.N., R.N.C., B.S.N., M.S.N.

Loyola University, Marcella Niehoff School of Nursing
Chicago, Illinois

Sherrilyn Coffman, R.N., B.S.N., M.S.N., D.N.S.

Florida Atlantic University College of Nursing
Boca Raton, Florida

Marsha Dowell, R.N., B.S.N., M.S.N.

University of Virginia, School of Nursing
Charlottesville, Virginia

Leann Eaton, R.N., B.S.N., M.S.N.

Jewish Hospital School of Nursing
St Louis, Missouri

Patricia R. Teasley, R.N., B.S.N., M.S.N., C.S.

Southern Union State Junior College
Valley, Alabama

Mary Crosley, R.N., B.S., M.S.

Suffolk County Community College
Brentwood, New York

**Teresa Marie Dobrzykowski, R.N., A.S.N., B.S.N.,
M.S.N.**

Indiana University at South Bend
South Bend, Indiana

Michael Dreyer, R.N., B.S.N., M.N.

LaSalle University, School of Nursing
Philadelphia, Pennsylvania

**JoAnn Schmidt-Festa, R.N.C., A.A.S., B.S., M.S.,
Ph.D.**

Nassau Community College
Garden City, New York

Bernadette Kahler, R.N., B.S.N., M.N.

Kansas Newman College
Wichita, Kansas

Ayda G. Nambayan, R.N., O.C.N., B.S.N., M.Ed.

University of Alabama at Birmingham School of
    Nursing
Birmingham, Alabama

Mary H. West, R.N., C.C.N., M.S.

Bob Jones University
Greenville, South Carolina

JoAnn Blake, R.N., B.S., M.S., Ph.D.

Prairie View A & M University College of Nursing
Houston, Texas

**Teresa S. Burckhalter, R.N., B.S.N., M.S.N., Cert.
Psych-Mental Health Nurse**

Technical College of the Low Country
Beaufort, South Carolina

Dorothy B. Lary, R.N., C.S., B.S.N., M.S.N.

Louisiana College
Pineville, Louisiana

Joan Cerniglia-Lowensen, R.N., B.S.N., M.S.N.

Union Memorial Hospital School of Nursing
Baltimore, Maryland

Rita Black Monsen, R.N., B.S.N., M.P.H., M.S.N., D.S.N.

Henderson State University
Arkadelphia, Arkansas

Anna P. Moore, R.N., B.S.N., M.S.

Petersburg General Hospital School of Nursing
Petersburg, Virginia

Ann T. Muller, R.N., B.S., M.Ed., Ph.D.

Private Practice
Dallas, Texas

Janice J. Rumfelt, R.N., B.S.N., M.S.N., Ed.D.

Southern Illinois University at Edwardsville School of
    Nursing
Edwardsville, Illinois

Phyllis Portnoy Cohen, R.N., R.N.C., M.S.

Long Island Jewish Medical Center
Division of OB/GYN
New Hyde Park, New York

Penelope L. Daniels, R.N., C.S., A.D.N.S.,B.S., B.S.N., M.S.

St. Mary's Hospital School of Nursing
Huntington, West Virginia

Shirley Ann Dufresne, R.N., B.S., M.S.N.

University of Massachusetts
North Dartmouth, Massachusetts

Carmel A. Esposito, R.N., B.S.N., M.S.N., Ed.D.

Ohio Valley Hospital School of Nursing
Steubenville, Ohio

Susan V. Gille, R.N., B.S.N., M.S.N., M.S.P.H., Ph.D.

Missouri Western State College
St. Joseph, Missouri

Caroline H. Hollshwandner, R.N., B.S.N., M.A., Ph.D.

Allentown College of St. Francis de Sales
Center Valley, Pennslyvania

Sharon Isaac, R.N., B.S.N., M.S.N., Ed.D.

University of Indianapolis, School of Nursing
Indianapolis, Indiana

Frances S. Izzo, R.N., A.A.S., B.S.N., M.S.N.

Nassau Community College
Garden City, New York

M. Susan Jones, R.N., B.S.N., M.S.N.

Western Kentucky University
Bowling Green, Kentucky

Christina Algiere Kasprisin, R.N., M.S.

University of Vermont School of Nursing
Burlington, Vermont

Elaine M. Kelter, R.N., B.S.N., M.S.

New England Baptist Hospital School of Nursing
Boston, Massachusetts

Shelia Marie Manis Kyle, R.N., A.S.N., B.S.N., M.S., M.S.N.

St. Mary's Hospital School of Nursing
Huntington, West Virginia

Joanne Lavin, R.N., B.S.N., M.S., M.Ed., Ed.D

Kingsborough Community College
Brooklyn, New York

Cecilia Mukai, R.N., B.S., M.S.N.

University of Hawaii at Hilo
Hilo, Hawaii

Ann D. Sprengel, R.N., B.S.N., M.S.N.

Southeast Missouri State University
Cape Girardeau, Missouri

Kathryn Sullivan, R.N., B.S.N., M.A., M.S.N., Ph. D., C.N.A.A.

Research College of Nursing
Kansas City, Missouri

Cecilia M. Tiller, R.N., B.S.N., M.N., D.S.N.

Medical College of Georgia School of Nursing
Augusta, Georgia

Janet R. Weber, R.N., B.S.N., M.S.N.

Southeast Missouri State University
Cape Girardeau, Missouri

Deborah Williams, R.N., A.S., B.A., M.S.N.

Western Kentucky University
Bowling Green, Kentucky

Frances A. Wollner, R.N., B.S., B.S.N., M.N.

Grand Island, New York

Preface

For almost 15 years MOSBY'S *AssessTest* has been helping students prepare for licensure. The National Council Licensure Examination for Registered Nurses (NCLEX-RN) in the United States and the Nurse Registration-Licensure Examination in Canada are based on normally encountered nursing situations that cross clinical disciplines. MOSBY'S *AssessTest* has been designed to assist nursing students to prepare for these examinations by evaluating their level of knowledge and providing feedback on clinical areas that may need further study. With the change in the NCLEX-RN to computerized adaptive testing (CAT), faculty and students need the benefits offered by the *AssessTest* now more than ever. These benefits provide both institutional and individual feedback that evaluates students' comprehension and assists faculty to evaluate specific curriculum content.

The 1998 *AssessTest* reflects the new NCLEX-CAT Examination. Approximately two-thirds of the students taking the NCLEX-RN pass or fail after 75 questions, the minimum number of questions every candidate must complete. *AssessTest*, therefore, includes four content-integrated tests of 75 questions each. Dividing the 300 questions into these four tests gives students a feel for the scope of content that will be covered on the NCLEX. It also allows faculty to administer each of the tests comfortably in a 90-minute block of time.

Like the NCLEX-RN, the multiple-choice questions in *AssessTest* offer four possible answers, and each question is independent of any other question. Each of the four tests covers nursing content equally in the core clinical areas of medicine, surgery, pediatrics, mental health, and childbearing and women's health. The test plan for *AssessTest* adheres to the guidelines for the components of Client Needs and Phases of the Nursing Process published by the National Council of State Boards of Nursing, Inc. in *NCLEX-RN Test Plan for the National Council Licensure Examination for Registered Nurses—Effective Date: October 1995.*

All 300 questions in *AssessTest* have been field tested by graduating students representing a broad geographic distribution and enrolled in baccalaureate, associate degree, and diploma nursing programs. This field testing ensures quality and validity of the questions. The questions reflect the latest knowledge, activities, procedures, medications, nursing diagnoses, and terminology encountered by the entry level nurse.

AssessTest provides each student with a computerized performance evaluation that includes:

- an overall summary of test results with comparison to the norm group, indicating how the student ranks compared to peers nationwide,
- a personal profile indicating clinical areas of greatest need for further study to help the student plan study time more effectively,
- a summary comparing performance to the norm group in nursing process, client needs, focus of care, and clinical area that assists in determining strengths and weaknesses, and
- a list of questions answered incorrectly and the response selected so the student can refer back to the test and review mistakes.

Each student also receives a booklet containing answers and rationales for every question on the test, which promotes further learning and understanding by explaining why the correct option was correct and why the other three were not correct. *MOSBY'S AssessTest* is a valuable diagnostic tool that provides extensive feedback on performance and makes even incorrect selections a learning opportunity.

The institutional profile is available to schools with 10 or more participants and is provided when answer sheets for the entire group are submitted for processing in a single batch. The extensive institutional analysis assists faculty in preparing their students for the examination and in evaluating the school's curriculum. The evaluative feedback for an institution:

- summarizes and compares the group's scores to the RN norm group and program-specific norm group so faculty can determine how students rank among peers,
- graphically summarizes performance overall and in nursing process, clinical area, focus of care, and client needs, which helps identify strengths and weaknesses of curriculum,
- provides a summary of group performance compared with both norm groups to assist faculty in curriculum evaluation,

- analyzes the group's performance by clinical areas for nursing process, focus of care, and client needs, which assists faculty in determining strengths and weaknesses of curriculum,
- includes the percentage of students choosing the correct answer for each question, which assists faculty in identifying specific questions their students found difficult,
- includes a student roster indicating the percent correct and percentile ranking relative to the RN norm group, assisting faculty in identifying students who need special help, and
- provides faculty a comparison of scores with last year's test that enables them to evaluate the consistency of student performance and curriculum.

It is readily apparent that the extensive analysis, statistics, and comparisons offered by *MOSBY'S AssessTest* can best be achieved using a standardized test. The nursing content that is tested and the structure of the questions all parallel the NCLEX-RN, providing a highly effective evaluation of students' readiness for the examination.

We would like to take this opportunity to thank Loren S. Wilson, our Editor, and Glenn Floyd, our Developmental Editor, for their management of our project; Billi Carcheri for her coordination of field testing and for her diligence in the preparation of our manuscript; our contributors and consultants; the students who participated in the field testing ventures; the proctors who administered the field tests; and our families for their support and sacrifice.

We sincerely hope that the *AssessTest* experience is challenging and beneficial to you. Good luck!

THE EDITORS

Contents

Introduction

WHAT IS *AssessTest*?

AssessTest is a computer-scored, multiple-choice examination designed to test essential nursing knowledge and evaluate ability to apply that knowledge to various clinical situations. The extensive computer analysis of your performance, which is the most outstanding feature of this test, will help you design effective and efficient plans for further study and review. Identification of your own specific strengths and weaknesses ought to eliminate much of the anxiety connected with deciding what material to study by giving you a sense of direction and a means of setting priorities. Designed to reflect the broad scope of basic nursing knowledge, *AssessTest* can be used for preparation and review in a variety of situations such as preparing for licensure examination, general evaluation for practicing nurses, review for nurses returning to work after an absence, or foreign-student preparation for qualifying examinations.

AssessTest consists of four randomly selected, content-integrated tests totaling 300 questions. Organized in a nursing process framework, the questions are constructed to reflect nursing situations that cross clinical disciplines. Clients rarely present an isolated health problem, and the nurse must be able to respond to individual needs regardless of the clinical area or diagnosis. The test requires you to respond to common human needs as well as to specific needs associated with given health problems.

CATEGORIES OF ABILITIES MEASURED BY *AssessTest*

Every question on *AssessTest* has been classified in each of five categories of abilities: (1) nursing behavior (phase of the nursing process), (2) clinical area, (3) client needs, (4) focus of care, and (5) category of concern.

Because *AssessTest* is an evaluative study tool, we have included nursing content to represent equally the clinical areas of medicine, surgery, pediatrics, mental health, and childbearing and women's health. This approach should be recognized as a deliberate variation from the NCLEX-RN. However, to reflect the types of questions the student will have to answer on the national examination in the categories of Nursing Process and Client Needs, we have selected questions that reflect the

percentages allocated to them in the NCLEX-RN Test Plan (October 1995). The questions used were randomly placed on the test after being selected from the pool of questions developed from the nationwide field testing. They reflect the latest activities, procedures, drugs, and nursing diagnoses.

Nursing behavior (phase of the nursing process)

In the United States and Canada, the licensure examinations are constructed in a nursing process framework. *AssessTest* also evaluates your ability to carry out the five components of the nursing process. These five components represent the various types of nursing behavior:

Assessment. The assessment phase of the nursing process involves gathering subjective and objective data about the client's health status from meaningful sources, grouping the data into categories, and communicating the information to others. The data base for making nursing decisions is determined through the assessing phase.

Analysis. In the analysis phase of the nursing process, the nurse interprets the data obtained during the assessment phase to identify the client's actual or potential health care needs and to formulate nursing diagnoses.

Planning. During the planning phase of the nursing process, the nurse designs strategies to correct, minimize, or prevent problems identified during the assessment and analysis phase; sets priorities for the problems diagnosed; develops both short-term and long-term goals with the client and/or client's family; establishes outcome criteria for nursing interventions; and writes the nursing care plan.

Implementation. In the implementation phase, the nurse initiates and completes the plan of care. The nurse may perform the care or assist, teach, counsel, or supervise the client, client's significant others, or other health team members to perform specific interventions based on the client's identified needs, diagnoses, priorities, and goals.

Evaluation. Through the evaluation component of the nursing process, the nurse determines the effectiveness of nursing intervention. In doing so, the nurse compares the actual outcomes with the expected outcomes to determine client compliance with and response to the intervention or therapy. The nurse uses the evaluation phase to identify whether the health care need still exists that would require modification of the plan, or whether new health care needs have developed that would require new interventions.

Clinical area

Each question in *AssessTest* has been coded as primarily pertaining to one of the clinical areas: **medical/ surgical nursing, childbearing and women's health nursing, pediatric nursing,** or **mental health nursing.**

Client needs

Client needs are those health care needs of the client that the nurse must address. The *AssessTest* evaluates four areas of client needs:

Support and promotion of physiologic and anatomic equilibrium. Meeting this need includes reducing risks that interfere with physiologic or anatomic integrity; promoting comfort and mobility; and providing basic care to assist, modify, or limit physiologic and anatomic adaptations.

An environment that is safe and conducive to effective therapeutic care. Addressing this need includes providing quality, goal-directed care that is coordinated, safe, and effective.

Education and other forms of health promotion to prevent, minimize, or correct actual or potential health problems. Fulfilling this need involves supporting optimal growth and development to provide for the achievement of the highest level of functioning. This level includes encouraging the use of support systems and self-care directed toward promoting the prevention, recognition, and treatment of disease throughout the life cycle.

Support and promotion of psychosocial and emotional equilibrium. Satisfying this need includes supporting individual emotional coping and adapting mechanisms to promote optimal emotional health while limiting or modifying those responses to crises that produce psychopathologic consequences.

Focus of care

In all nursing situations, real and hypothetical, there are factors that dictate a focus of care for the client, the family, and the community itself. This focus influences the nurse's actions and crosses the clinical areas, steps in the nursing process, client needs, and category of concern:

Acute Care. The focus of care is on clients in emergency, ambulatory, critical care, surgical, and emotional crisis situations

Community-based Care. The focus of care is on clients who are receiving care in a community setting and on the health of the community itself

Older Adult Care. The focus of care is on older adult clients with special age-related changes that may or may not be associated with their current health problems

Health Maintenance/Promotion. The focus of care is on helping clients achieve and maintain optimum health

Long-term Care. The focus of care is on helping clients adjust to long-term health problems that require changes in daily living practices and activities

Categories of concern

The categories of concern are indicators of the specific content areas within the broad clinical areas.

The following categories of concern are used in **medical/surgical** and **pediatric nursing:** blood and immunity, cardiovascular, drug-related responses, emotional needs related to health problems, endocrine, fluid and electrolyte, gastrointestinal, growth and development, integumentary, neuromuscular, reproductive and genitourinary, respiratory, and skeletal.

The following categories of concern are used in **childbearing and women's health nursing:** drug-related responses, emotional needs related to childbearing and women's health, healthy childbearing, high-risk maternal-fetal conditions affecting childbearing, high-risk neonate, normal neonate, reproductive choices, reproductive problems, and women's health.

The following categories of concern are used in **mental health nursing:** anxiety, somatoform, and dissociative disorders; crisis situations; dementia, delirium, and other cognitive disorders; disorders first evident before adulthood; disorders of mood; disorders of personality; drug-related responses; eating disorders; emotional problems related to physical health and childbearing; personality development; schizophrenic disorders; substance abuse; and therapeutic relationships.

HOW TO MAXIMIZE THE BENEFITS OF YOUR *AssessTest* EXPERIENCE

Use this opportunity to become "test wise."

Do you really know what a multiple-choice question is? Do you know how to read multiple-choice questions carefully? Do you know how to choose wisely among alternative answers to questions? Test-taking skills and techniques are not a substitute for good study habits or an adequate grasp of the content and abilities measured in an examination. If you have a thorough understanding of the knowledge measured in an examination, however, good test-taking skills will enhance your overall performance.

To become oriented to test-taking skills that you can use in taking examinations such as *AssessTest* or licensure examinations, you need to know something about the language of multiple-choice questions. The question in its entirety is called a test item. The portion of the test item that poses the question or problem is called the stem. Potential answers to the question or problem posed are called options. In well-constructed multiple-choice items there is only one correct answer among the options supplied; the incorrect options are called distractors. Look at the following item and see if you can correctly label the item components.

The first step in the nursing process is:
1. Planning
2. Analyzing
3. Evaluation
4. Assessment

In this sample item, option **4** is correct; options **1, 2,** and **3** are the distractors. In this example the stem is in the form of an incomplete sentence, and each of the options could complete it. Stems may also be stated as questions. For instance, the stem could have read: "What is the first step in the nursing process?"

Remember that test questions are meant to measure your nursing knowledge. The items may be easy to read, but the answers to questions are not intended to be readily apparent. The questions draw on your ability to apply nursing knowledge from a variety of sources.

The following test-taking methods can increase your probability of choosing the correct answer to a question.

Read questions carefully. Scores on written tests are strongly affected by reading ability. In answering a test item, you should begin by carefully reading the stem and then asking yourself the following questions:

What is the question really asking?

Are there any key words?

What information relevant to answering this question is included in the stem?

How would I ask this question in my own words?

How would I answer this question in my own words?

After you have answered these questions, carefully read the options and then ask yourself the following questions:

Is there an option that is similar to the one I thought of?

Is this option the best, most complete answer to the question?

Deal with the question as it is stated, without reading anything into it or making assumptions about it. Answer the question asked, not the one you would like to answer. For simple recall items the self-questioning process will usually be completed quickly. For more complex items the self-questioning process may take longer, but it should assist you in clarifying the item and selecting the best response.

Eliminate clearly wrong or incorrect answers. Eliminate clearly incorrect, inappropriate, and unlikely answers to the question asked in the stem. By systematically eliminating distractors that are unlikely in the con-

text of a given question, you increase the probability of selecting the correct answer. Eliminating obvious distractors also allows you more time to focus on the options that appear to be potentially sound answers to the question. Consider the following example:

The phases of the nursing process include:
1. Assessment, analysis, implementation, evaluation
2. Knowledge, comprehension, application, analysis
3. Planning, analysis, assessment, comprehension
4. Medical/surgical nursing, pediatric nursing, psychiatric nursing

Options **2** and **3** contain both cognitive levels and phases of the nursing process, thus eliminating them from consideration. Option **4** is clearly inappropriate, as the choices are all clinical areas. Option **1** contains four of the five phases of the nursing process. Therefore option **1** is correct. By reducing the plausible options, you reduce the material to consider and increase the probability of selecting the correct option.

Identify similar options. When an item contains two or more options that are very similar in meaning, the successful test taker knows that all are correct, in which case it is a poor question, or that none is correct, which is more likely to be the case. The correct option will usually either include all the similar options or exclude them entirely.

In teaching new diabetics about their condition, it is important to focus on:
1. Dietary modifications
2. Use of exchange lists
3. Use of sugar substitutes
4. Their present understanding of diabetes

Options **1, 2,** and **3** deal only with the diabetic diet, involving no other aspect of diabetic teaching; it is impossible to select the most correct option because each represents an equally plausible, though limited, answer to the question. Option **4** is the best choice because it includes the other three options and is most complete. It therefore allows the other three options to be excluded as answers.

A child's intelligence is influenced by:
1. A variety of factors
2. Heredity and environment
3. Environment and experience
4. Education and economic factors

The most correct answer is option **1**. It includes the material covered by the other options, eliminating the need for an impossible choice, as each of the other options is only partially correct.

Identify answer (option) components. When an answer contains two or more parts, you can reduce the number of potentially correct answers by identifying one part as incorrect.

The nurse is aware that the signs of pregnancy-induced hypertension would include:
1. *Proteinuria, hypotension, weight gain*
2. *Proteinuria, hypertension, weight gain*
3. *Ketonuria, hypotension, pitting edema*
4. *Ketonuria, hypertension, physiologic edema*

If you know, for instance, that pregnancy-induced hypertension does in fact cause hypertension, you can eliminate options **1** and **3** from consideration. If you know that pregnancy-induced hypertension causes protein in the urine rather than ketones you can eliminate option **4**. Therefore option **2** is correct.

Identify specific determiners. When the options of a test item contain words that are identical or similar to words in the stem, the alert test taker recognizes the similarities as clues about the likely answer to the question. The stem word that clues you to a similar word in the option or that limits potential options is known as a specific determiner.

The government agency responsible for administering the nursing practice act in each state is the:
1. *Board of nursing*
2. *Board of regents*
3. *State nurses' association*
4. *State hospital association*

Options **1** and **3** contain the closely related words nurse and nursing. The word *nursing*, used both in the stem and in option **1**, is a clue to the correct answer.

Identify words in the options that are closely associated with words in the stem. Be alert to words in the options that may be closely associated with but not identical to a word or words in the stem.

When a person develops symptoms of physical illness for which psychogenic factors act as causative agents, the resulting illness is classified as:
1. *Dissociative*
2. *Compensatory*
3. *Psychophysiologic*
4. *Reaction formation*

Option **3** should strike you as a likely answer, as it combines physical and psychologic factors, like those referred to in the stem.

Be alert to relevant information from earlier questions. Occasionally, information from one question may provide you with a clue for answering future questions.

A client has a nasogastric tube inserted after surgery. The nurse is aware that gastric suction can result in excessive loss of:
1. *Protein enzymes*
2. *Energy carbohydrates*
3. *Water and electrolytes*
4. *Vitamins and minerals*

If you know that the correct answer is option **3**, it may help you to answer a later question, which asks:
Critical assessment of a client while an intestinal tube is draining should include observation for:
1. *Edema*
2. *Nausea*
3. *Belching*
4. *Dehydration*

The correct answer is option **4**. If you knew that excessive loss of water and electrolytes from nasogastric or intestinal suction may lead to dehydration, you could have used the clue provided in the earlier question to assist you in answering the later question.

Pay attention to specific details. The well-written multiple-choice question is precisely stated, providing you with only the information needed to make the question or problem clear and specific. Careful reading of details in the stem can provide you with important clues to the correct option.

A male client is told that he will no longer be able to ingest alcohol if he wants to live. To effect a change in the client's behavior while he is in the hospital, the nurse should attempt to:
1. *Help the client set short-term dietary goals*
2. *Discuss his hopes and dreams for the future*
3. *Discuss the pathophysiology of the liver with him*
4. *Withhold approval until he agrees to stop drinking*

The specific clause to effect a change in the client's behavior while he is in the hospital is critical. Option **2** is not really related to the client's alcoholism. Option **3** may be part of educating the alcoholic client, but you would not expect a behavioral change observable in the hospital to emerge from this discussion. Option **4** rejects the client as well as the client's behavior instead of only the client's behavior. Option **1**, the correct answer, could result in an observable behavioral change while the client is hospitalized; for example, the client could define ways to achieve short-term goals relating to diet and alcohol while in the hospital.

Identify key words. Certain key words in the stem, the options, or both should alert you to the need for caution in choosing your answer. Some of these key words are *all, never, only, must, no, none, always, except,* and *every.* These are strong words. They place special limitations and qualifications on potentially correct answers.

All of the following are services of the National Kidney Foundation except:
1. *Public education programs*
2. *Research about kidney disease*
3. *Fund-raising affairs for research activities*
4. *Identification of potential transplant recipients*

The stem contains two key words: *all* and *except*. They limit the choice of a correct answer to the one option that does not represent a service of the National Kidney Foundation. When *except*, *not*, or a phrase such as *all but one of the following* appears in the stem, the inappropriate option is the correct answer; in this instance, option **4**. Also be on guard when you see one of the key words in an option; it may limit the contexts in which such an option would be correct.

If the options in an item do not seem to make sense because more than one is correct, reread the question; you may have missed some key words in the stem.

The nurse teaches a client with diabetes mellitus how to perform foot care. The nurse would recognize that further teaching was necessary when the client states:
1. *"I will visit my podiatrist every 6 weeks."*
2. *"I will check my feet daily for signs of pressure."*
3. *"I will wash and gently dry my feet at least twice a day."*
4. *"I will wear only nylon or nylon and cotton–mixed socks."*

In this question the stem is really asking which response by the client is incorrect and needs to be changed by further education. Options **1**, **2**, and **3** demonstrate an appropriate level of understanding, whereas option **4** is incorrect and demonstrates a need for further teaching.

Watch for grammatical inconsistencies. If one or more of the options is not grammatically consistent with the stem, the alert test taker can frequently eliminate these distractors. When the stem is in the form of an incomplete sentence, each option should complete the sentence in a grammatically correct way. The correct option must be consistent with the form of the question. If the question demands a response in the singular, plural options usually can be safely eliminated.

The nurse is aware that initiating communication with a client who is deaf will be facilitated by:
1. *The use of gestures*
2. *Facing the client while speaking*
3. *Find out if the client has a hearing aid*
4. *Speaking loudly often helps clients hear*

Options **3** and **4** do not complete the sentence in a grammatically consistent way and can be safely eliminated, leaving the choice between options **1** and **2**. Option **1** may help once the client and nurse have established a nonverbal mode of communication, but gestures can frequently be misunderstood initially, leaving option **2** as the best choice.

Make educated guesses. On the computerized NCLEX, you will not be able to go on to the next question until an answer is selected for the present question. You can generally eliminate one or more of the distrac-tors by using partial knowledge and the methods just listed. The elimination process increases your chances of selecting the correct option from those remaining. Elimination of two distractors on a four-option multiple-choice item increases your probability of selecting the correct answer from 25% to 50%. First use educated guesses, then move to pure guessing. You have at least a 1 in 4 (25%) chance of guessing the correct answer.

Use the rules of test wisdom

- Study! There is no escape! All the test-taking skills and techniques will be of little use if you do not have a good grasp of the content to be tested.
- Follow all written or oral directions for taking the test.
- Read carefully and think about what you read.
- Remember that every word in a question matters. Attend to detail.
- Answer the question asked.
- Put questions and answers in your own words to test your comprehension.
- Read each option carefully and compare options, looking for similarities and conflicts among them.
- Eliminate obviously incorrect options quickly so you can spend time on more plausible ones.
- Relate options to the question asked.
- Look for clues in the question that might lead you to the correct option.
- Watch for key words such as *all*, *never*, and *only* in both the questions and the options.
- Assess grammatical and logical consistency between the question and each option. Eliminate options that are inconsistent.
- Attempt to recall clues from previous questions.
- Be aware of cultural differences and moral biases, but do not base your answers on your personal beliefs and practices.
- Avoid selecting answers that reflect specific hospital policies, rules, or regulations.
- Be alert for questions that require you to determine priorities among four plausible options. State criteria for determining priorities to yourself.
- Make educated guesses.
- Select the option that provides the most complete, appropriate answer to the question.
- Stay with your first answer unless you have a very specific reason to change it.

Use this opportunity to learn how to manage your test-taking time

Because many examinations have specified time lim-its (even the NCLEX/CAT has a maximum time of 5 hours), you will need to pace yourself during the testing period and work as quickly and accurately as possible. On examinations where the exact number of questions and the allotted time is known, it is helpful to estimate the time that can be spent on each item and still complete the examination in the allotted time. Obtain this figure by dividing the testing time by the number of items on the test. For example, with a 75-minute testing period and 75 items, an average of 1 minute per item will be the appropriate pace.

Although certain questions will be more difficult than others and will require more time, spending too much time on these difficult items may compromise your overall score. On the *AssessTest* you can make a mark next to the item you cannot answer and go on. After you have answered all the questions you can answer easily, return to the marked items. Be sure to erase any extraneous marks near your answers. If time remains, it is useful to review all your answers, making sure you have marked them correctly.

Note: For the NCLEX-RN CAT, you will be unable to return to any previous question, and every question must be answered before moving on.

Do not be pressured into finishing early. Do not rush! Typically, students who achieve higher scores use all the time available.

Use this opportunity to build your test-taking confidence

You should feel confident and competent if you have studied and reviewed the content to be tested and you are armed with methods for reading and answering questions. Questions that seem complicated at first glance can often be answered with the "educated guess." Remain calm and confident. Your emotional state is vitally important when thinking about, preparing for, and taking any test. Think positively.

Use the *AssessTest* as a learning experience

The *AssessTest* is a valuable evaluating tool designed to test your level of knowledge. However, it is equally as valuable in providing information from incorrect answers. By studying the rationales for the incorrect selections, you will have an excellent opportunity to learn from your mistakes. In addition, the computer analysis of your performance that you receive will identify areas of strength and weakness, information that will assist you when focusing study time.

COMPUTER EVALUATION

After your completed answer sheet has been processed and scored, you will receive a computerized evaluation of your test results. The evaluation will provide specific data regarding your overall performance and your performance in each of the categories measured by *AssessTest*. You will also receive a booklet of "Answers and Rationales" that has been designed to help the testee understand why the correct answer was correct and the reason each of the incorrect answers was incorrect for each question on the *AssessTest*. The booklet also indicates the classifications for each question.

The introduction to this booklet explains how to interpret your computer analysis and how best to use the data on the report to design a personal study plan. Using this information along with the questions in the *AssessTest* and the "Answers and Rationales" booklet will help you learn from your mistakes and make the most of your *AssessTest* experience.

AssessTest

DIRECTIONS FOR TAKING *AssessTest*

To gain the maximum benefit from this experience, it is vital that you follow *precisely* and *completely* the directions for taking the examination and returning the answer sheet. The personal computer analysis you receive will give you a true picture of your abilities if you have taken the test under conditions that are as controlled as possible and if your answers reflect your best efforts. Be sure that you have not overlooked or misunderstood any test directions and that the rules and procedures of the examination are absolutely clear to you before beginning.

Materials needed

You will need the following materials:
1. Your test manual
2. Answer sheet (included with manual)
3. A number 2 (soft lead) pencil (Do not use a ballpoint pen, colored lead, or any other type of writing instrument. The tests are machine scored, and only answers marked with a soft-lead pencil will be recorded.)
4. An eraser

Time needed

There are four comprehensive tests. Each test consists of 75 questions. It is assumed that you will use about 1 minute per question. Allow 75 minutes for each comprehensive test.

How to take the test

1. Read each question *carefully.*
2. Go through the test you are working on once, answering the questions you feel sure about first.
3. Go back over the test a second time and answer the remaining questions. Answer *all* the questions. If you must guess, eliminate the obviously incorrect answers first and base your guess on the remaining alternatives. You will receive feedback based on the responses you select.
4. Because the computer printout will keep track of *only* the questions you answered incorrectly, you should circle your answers directly on the test booklet as well as marking your answer sheet. By circling the answers in the test booklet, you will have a record of all of your responses. *The analysis you receive will not include a record of your correct responses.*

NOTE: Your score on *AssessTest* is based on the number of questions you answer correctly. The number of questions missed is subtracted from the total number of questions (300) to determine your score. Because *AssessTest* is designed to help you identify your strengths and weaknesses, it is to your advantage to answer all the questions. Be sure you understand the grading system when taking examinations. Guide your test-taking approach accordingly.

How to complete the answer sheet

Read these directions carefully *before* filling out the answer sheet. Use only a number 2 (soft lead) pencil. Make heavy, black marks. Erase thoroughly if you change an answer. Record answers in designated spaces only. Do not make any other marks on the answer sheet.

Side 1 (personal data)

Please answer all questions and print clearly.
1. *Your name.* Print your name in the row of empty boxes provided, skipping one space between words. As you enter each letter, darken the oval with the corresponding printed letter in the column directly below it. Do not make dots, crosses, circles, Xs, or lines; fill in only a single oval for each letter.
2. *Your mailing address.* Fill in the boxes as you did with your name, marking appropriate letters or numbers beneath those you have entered. Use the following abbreviations in the street number and name and city or town as necessary:

APARTMENT	APT
AVENUE	AVE
BOULEVARD	BLVD
BOX	BX
CENTER	CTR
CIRCLE	CIR
CITY	CTY
COLLEGE	COL
COMMUNITY	CMTY

COUNTY	CNTY	CALIFORNIA	CA
COURT	CT	COLORADO	CO
DRIVE	DR	CONNECTICUT	CT
EAST	E	DELAWARE	DE
FLOOR	FLR	DISTRICT OF COLUMBIA	DC
FORT	FT	FLORIDA	FL
GARDEN	GDN	GEORGIA	GA
GENERAL	GEN	HAWAII	HI
HEALTH	HLTH	IDAHO	ID
HEIGHTS	HTS	ILLINOIS	IL
HIGHWAY	HWY	INDIANA	IN
HOSPITAL	HSP	IOWA	IA
INSTITUTE	INST	KANSAS	KS
JUNCTION	JCT	KENTUCKY	KY
LAKE	LK	LOUISIANA	LA
LANE	LN	MAINE	ME
MEDICAL	MED	MARYLAND	MD
MEMORIAL	MEM	MASSACHUSETTS	MA
MOUNT	MT	MICHIGAN	MI
MOUNTAIN	MT	MINNESOTA	MN
NORTH	N	MISSISSIPPI	MS
PARK	PK	MISSOURI	MO
PARKWAY	PKWY	MONTANA	MT
PIKE	PI	NEBRASKA	NE
PLACE	PL	NEVADA	NV
POINT	PT	NEW HAMPSHIRE	NH
PORT	PT	NEW JERSEY	NJ
POST OFFICE	PO	NEW MEXICO	NM
REGIONAL	REG	NEW YORK	NY
ROAD	RD	NORTH CAROLINA	NC
ROUTE	RT	NORTH DAKOTA	ND
SCHOOL	SCH	OHIO	OH
SERVICE	SVC	OKLAHOMA	OK
SOUTH	S	OREGON	OR
STATION	STA	PENNSYLVANIA	PA
STREET	ST	RHODE ISLAND	RI
TECHNICAL	TECH	SOUTH CAROLINA	SC
TERRACE	TR	SOUTH DAKOTA	SD
TRAIL	TR	TENNESSEE	TN
TRAILER	TRLR	TEXAS	TX
TURNPIKE	TPKE	UTAH	UT
UNIVERSITY	UNIV	VERMONT	VT
WARD	WD	VIRGINIA	VA
WAY	WY	WASHINGTON	WA
WEST	W	WEST VIRGINIA	WV
		WISCONSIN	WI
		WYOMING	WY
		PUERTO RICO	PR
		VIRGIN ISLANDS	VI
		ALBERTA	AB
		BRITISH COLUMBIA	BC
		MANITOBA	MB
		NEW BRUNSWICK	NB

In the two boxes labeled *State* or *Province* enter one of the following abbreviations and fill in the ovals corresponding to the letters you have entered:

ALABAMA	AL
ALASKA	AK
ARIZONA	AZ
ARKANSAS	AR

NORTHWEST TERRITORIES	NT
NOVA SCOTIA	NS
ONTARIO	ON
PRINCE EDWARD ISLAND	PE
PROVINCE OF QUEBEC	PQ
SASKATCHEWAN	SK
YUKON TERRITORY	YT
LABRADOR	LB
NEWFOUNDLAND	NF
NOT LISTED	NL

Mark the appropriate space in the box labeled *Country of Current Mailing Address.*

3. *Demographic questions.* Answer all questions on the lower part of the form. Select only one response for each question (the one that is most nearly correct). This information will be used only for statistical purposes and will in no way affect your test results.
4. *School name.* If you are still in school or have recently graduated and have not yet taken the licensure examination, indicate your nursing school. If you are a licensed nurse in practice, indicate the name of the hospital or institution with which you are affiliated. If you are taking the test as a required part of a review course not conducted by your nursing school, indicate the name of the course.
5. *Date.* Fill in the date on which you complete the test.

If your state or province is not listed and you enter NL in the boxes, complete your mailing address on Side 2 of your answer sheet.

Side 2 (answer sheet)

You are now ready to begin the first test. Fill out the answer sheet as follows:
1. Print your address at the top of the answer sheet in the spaces provided.
2. Turn to Comprehensive Examination 1 in the booklet.
3. Start with the space marked 1 under Test 1 on your answer sheet (Side 2). Mark only one answer per question. Use a number 2 (soft lead) pencil. Make heavy, dark marks. Erase changes completely. Be sure you put your answers in the correct spaces on your answer sheet. Check question numbers as you go.
4. Complete all four tests. Try to finish at least one whole test at a sitting.

Returning the answer sheet

When you have completed all four tests, enter the date of completion on Side 1. Return the completed answer sheet to your instructor, who will mail all documents for scoring. **Do not mail your own answer sheet unless you are taking this test as an individual.**

DIRECTIONS FOR GROUP ADMINISTRATION OF *AssessTest*

To obtain a statistical summary of group performance, your group must include 10 or more participants. You may divide the test administration into whatever time periods are convenient for you, but it is suggested that at least one test be completed per sitting. Each test requires 75 minutes for completion. The answer sheet is to be filled in as described on pp. 16 to 18.

To obtain the computer profile of your group's performance, you *must* send all of the students' answer sheets in for scoring at one time. Answer sheets should be mailed first class in *one* envelope. A pre-addressed envelope is provided with your order. Answer sheets should be stacked, unclipped, unstapled, and unfolded.

Mail to:

Mosby's RN *AssessTest*
Professional Testing Corporation
1211 Avenue of the Americas
15th Floor
New York, NY 10036

Please be sure the envelope bears adequate postage.

A cover sheet must be completed and placed on top of the answer sheets. A cover sheet is provided with your order. If it has been misplaced, use the copy on p. 19. Please fill out the cover sheet completely and neatly. Be sure to indicate the type of program: diploma, associate degree, or baccalaureate. *All the tests for your group must be returned together.* This is the only way that you can obtain your institutional profile with the summary document of your group's performance. The individual test results may be returned *either* to your institution or to the individual student. **If you do not indicate where individual results should be sent, they will be mailed to the institution.** The institutional summary will be mailed to the institution. Please keep in mind that no test results will be mailed before April 1. Any questions should be directed to Mosby-Year Book, Inc., St. Louis, Missouri. Write or call toll-free (800) 633-6699.

Comprehensive examination 1

1. A client who is a gestational diabetic now requires insulin for glucose control. To address the nursing diagnosis of knowledge deficit, the nurse should teach the client that:
   1. Hyperglycemic reactions have a sudden onset
   2. Hypoglycemic reactions are caused by too much insulin
   3. Hypoglycemic reactions are characterized by flushed, dry skin
   4. Hyperglycemic reactions are associated with nervousness and shakiness

2. When taking a client's blood pressure during a community screening program, it is important that the nurse:
   1. Immediately inflate the cuff back over the number in question if uncertain of a reading
   2. Wrap the cuff loosely to avoid a snug fit and possible vasoconstriction before the actual measurement
   3. Talk with the client while wrapping and inflating the cuff and allow the client to talk during the actual measurement to promote relaxation
   4. Inflate the cuff to a pressure 30 mm higher than anticipated or the last systolic reading and release the pressure at a rate of 5 mm per second

3. A client had a transuretheral resection of the prostate (TURP) and has a continuous bladder irrigation (CBI). Four hours after surgery the nurse observes that the urine is bright red with numerous clots and that the client is in pain. The vital signs are BP 90/60, T 99.6° F (37.6° C) orally, P 108, R 24. The primary nursing diagnosis is:
   1. Impaired gas exchange related to pain
   2. Fluid volume deficit related to blood loss
   3. Hyperthermia related to inflammatory response
   4. Fluid volume excess related to CBI irrigating fluid

4. An appropriate nursing action to treat a client who is having an insulin reaction is:
   1. Give the client one cup of milk and notify the physician
   2. Monitor vital signs and urinary output and notify the physician
   3. Assess for symptoms specific to the client's hypoglycemia and chart these accurately
   4. Test for glucose with a glucometer and give insulin according to the sliding-scale order

5. A 65-year-old client with cancer of the larynx undergoes radiation therapy for 5 weeks prior to a neck dissection and tumor excision. When the client asks how long the postsurgical recovery time will be, the nurse should reply:
   1. "I really don't know. It is different for everyone but speak to your surgeon."
   2. "Your medicare insurance will cover the whole length of your stay, so don't worry."
   3. "You shouldn't worry about how long you are going to stay; you should focus on getting better."
   4. "It may be a little longer than average; the radiation you received sometimes delays tissue healing."

6. A preterm infant's axillary temperature is 98° F (36.7° C). The nurse should plan to care for this infant by:
   1. Turning up the temperature of the Isolette
   2. Maintaining the neutral thermal environment
   3. Initiating a sepsis workup due to a subnormal temperature
   4. Placing the infant on a radiant warmer to reduce air conduction.

7. A vaginal examination is not performed on a client with a placenta previa because it might:
   1. Cause profuse bleeding
   2. Rupture the membranes
   3. Increase the risk of infection
   4. Stimulate harder contractions

8. Ten days following replacement of an arthritic hip, an 80-year-old client is having watery stools almost constantly. The nurse should first:
   1. Increase fluids
   2. Check for a fecal impaction
   3. Request an order for Kaopectate
   4. Discontinue the prescribed stool softener

9. A 15-year-old male adolescent is struggling with a young sister's diagnosis of cancer. The nurse could best support him by:
   1. Encouraging him to join a support group
   2. Suggesting he take up sports to work out his feelings
   3. Advising him to help his sister with prescribed therapies
   4. Telling him to express his feelings away from the home environment

10. Baseline pulmonary function tests are done on an 8-year-old, which include an assessment of arterial blood gases. The findings that are within the normal range for this age are:
    1. PO_2 30 and CO_2 10
    2. PO_2 60 and CO_2 30
    3. PO_2 90 and CO_2 50
    4. PO_2 95 and CO_2 40

11. A nursery nurse observes that a 30-minute-old newborn just admitted to the nursery has a discharge coming from both eyes. The best nursing intervention for this infant is to:
    1. Call the physician to report the eye discharge
    2. Culture the eye discharge and send it to the laboratory
    3. Place the infant on sepsis precautions and notify the obstetrician
    4. Check the infant's record to see if ophthalmic antibiotics were given

12. An infant born at 28 weeks gestation is experiencing periods of apnea and bradycardia, is grunting, and has substernal and intercostal retractions. The nurse will establish the nursing diagnosis as:
    1. Decreased cardiac output related to prematurity
    2. Ineffective airway clearance related to immature lungs
    3. Impaired gas exchange related to decreased surfactant
    4. Ineffective breathing pattern related to meconium aspiration

13. A client with Type 1 diabetes mellitus delivers a 10 lb 2 oz (4593 g) baby. Priority nursing care would include assessment of the newborn for:
    1. Hip abduction
    2. Urinary output
    3. Gestational age
    4. Abdominal girth

14. When planning for discharge of a client with a slowly healing abdominal surgical wound, the foods that are most important for the nurse to recommend are:
    1. Acid-ash fruits
    2. Lean-cut meats
    3. Low-fat dairy products
    4. High-cellulose vegetables

15. Following a kidney transplantation, a client gains two pounds of body weight in one day. The additional finding that most supports the nurse's suspicion of kidney rejection is:
    1. Vague, persistent epigastric pain
    2. A subnormal serum creatinine level
    3. Development of urinary incontinence
    4. Above normal blood pressure readings

16. A client is in the early postoperative period following removal of a large tumor of the left cerebrum when the nurse observes the client's spouse repositioning the client in bed. It would be most appropriate for the nurse to instruct the spouse to:
    1. Keep the bed flat until cerebral bleeding has been controlled
    2. Avoid repositioning the client until the surgical wound is healed
    3. Carefully log roll the client in a right side-back-left side regimen
    4. Position the client on the right side or back but avoid the left side

17. When initially approaching a client who appears to be responding to auditory hallucinations, the nurse's most therapeutic response would be:
    1. "May I interrupt your conversation?"
    2. "Tell me about the conversation you are having."
    3. "I've noticed that you seem to be talking to someone."
    4. "You seem to be talking and there is no one else here."

18. A client, with a history of heavy alcohol use, whose last drink was 24 hours ago is seen in the emergency service. The client is oriented but is tremulous, weak, sweaty, and has some GI symptoms. This group of symptoms is typical of:
    1. Delirium tremens
    2. Korsakoff's syndrome
    3. Pathologic intoxication
    4. Alcohol withdrawal syndrome

19. A client is admitted with an antisocial personality disorder. The client is charming, friendly, and very social. The nurse would expect the client to demonstrate:
    1. Instability of mood
    2. Ritualistic behaviors
    3. Poor impulse control
    4. Appropriate interactions with staff and peers

23

20. To help a young couple with the grief work following the death of their 3-month-old son from SIDS, the nurse should:
    1. Leave them alone in a room so they can express their feelings privately
    2. Collect a very thorough health history on the baby to help in the diagnosis
    3. Facilitate their receiving an initial oral or written autopsy report as soon as possible
    4. Take the baby to the morgue right away so they are not reminded of what happened

21. A child with an antisocial personality disorder continues to exhibit poor academic performance. From the study of personality disorders the school nurse remembers that according to Freud:
    1. All behavior has meaning
    2. The prognosis for behavior change is excellent
    3. The behavior pattern of personality disorders is inherited
    4. Intense and unstable relationships are important to these people

22. When planning care for a client who is in Buck's traction, the nurse should be particularly alert for the development of:
    1. Swelling of the knee joint
    2. Excoriation of skin at the groin
    3. Spasms of the calf and foot muscles
    4. Plantar flexion and eversion of the foot

23. A client with carpal tunnel syndrome is being treated conservatively. Prescriptions include pain medications, a hand splint, and a steroid injection into the synovial area of the right carpal tunnel. Following the steroid injection, the nurse should instruct the client to:
    1. Use the hand splint to rest and protect the right hand
    2. Exercise by flexing, extending, and rotating the right hand
    3. Take the pain medication every 4 hours, even if the hand is not hurting
    4. Observe for occurrence of steroidal side effects such as weight gain and moon face

24. Four hours after a right radical neck dissection, a client begins to hemorrhage. The nurse's best action while waiting for the surgeon is to:
    1. Remove the dressing, replace it with a pressure dressing, and then go for help
    2. Stay with the client, apply pressure over the left carotid and internal jugular vessels

    3. Apply pressure over the dressings and over the right carotid and internal jugular vessels
    4. Stay with the client, remove the bloody dressing, and replace it with a pressure dressing

25. The nurse recognizes that a 12-year-old understands self-administration of Humulin N insulin when the child states:
    1. "I should insert the needle at a slight angle."
    2. "I should take my insulin 3 hours after meals."
    3. "I will inject my insulin into my arm every day."
    4. "My insulin should peak about 6 hours after I take it."

26. The nurse recognizes that the mother of a toddler with celiac disease understands the dietary restrictions when she states that she does not give her child any:
    1. Bread and pasta
    2. White rice and corn
    3. Potatoes and brown rice
    4. Lima beans and soybeans

27. When assessing the laboratory tests for a toddler with nephrotic syndrome, the nurse would expect to find:
    1. Anemia
    2. Hypernatremia
    3. Hypoalbuminemia
    4. Thrombocytopenia

28. An 80-year-old client, newly admitted to a long-term care facility, becomes confused regarding time and place. The nurse initiates a reality orientation program and, when the client's perceptions are contradicted, the client becomes belligerent during the session. At this point it is best for the nurse to:
    1. Request an order for a tranquilizer
    2. Continue to confront the client with reality
    3. Move the client to a different location in the facility
    4. Verbally express empathy with the client's misperceptions

29. A 13-year-old is admitted to an inpatient treatment center following a serious suicidal attempt. The nursing priority when planning the emergency care for this child would be:
    1. Physical safety of the child

24

2. Environmental safety of the child
3. Long-term goals to include better problem solving
4. Psychosocial assessment and history of the event

30. One week after starting fluphenazine decanoate (Prolixin Decanoate) therapy a client demonstrates muscle rigidity, stupor, incontinence, elevated serum creatine phosphokinase (CPK), hyperkalemia, high fever, tachycardia, and signs of renal failure. The nurse should immediately call the physician because these symptoms are indicative of:
1. Akinesia
2. Acute dystonia
3. Tardive dyskinesia
4. Neuroleptic malignant syndrome

31. To suction a client's tracheostomy, it would be most appropriate for the nurse to apply suction for:
1. 25 to 35 seconds while inserting the catheter and rotate the catheter 360°
2. 10 to 15 seconds while inserting the catheter and rotate the catheter 180°
3. 25 to 30 seconds while withdrawing the catheter and rotate the catheter 180°
4. 10 to 15 seconds while withdrawing the catheter and rotate the catheter 360°

32. A client who is on a mechanical respirator begins to fight the respirator. Pancuronium bromide (Pavulon) is ordered. This drug is classified as:
1. An antihistamine
2. An anticholinergic
3. A psychotherapeutic
4. A neuromuscular blocking agent

33. A client being weaned from the ventilator has arterial blood gases drawn. The results are: pH 7.31; PO_2 90; PCO_2 58; HCO_3 26. The nurse identifies this as uncompensated:
1. Metabolic acidosis
2. Metabolic alkalosis
3. Respiratory acidosis
4. Respiratory alkalosis

34. The assessment data of a child with acute lymphocytic leukemia (ALL) that would support a nursing diagnosis of high risk for injury (hemorrhage) related to interference with cell proliferation is:

1. Fatigue, lethargy, hematocrit 27%
2. Hemoglobin 9.2%, pallor, malaise
3. Petechiae, platelet count 45,000, bruising
4. Elevated temperature, WBC 4,000, diaphoresis

35. A child is receiving D5 ⅓ NS at 30 mL/hr IV. Using microdrip tubing, the nurse should make certain that the IV rate is set at:
1. 15 gtts/min
2. 30 gtts/min
3. 45 gtts/min
4. 60 gtts/min

36. A child with glomerulonephritis has a decreased urine output. The blood pressure, which has risen to 150/76, is being treated with hydralazine (Apresoline). Based on this information, the nurse plans a breakfast of:
1. Sausage, pancakes with syrup, and 8 ounces of milk
2. Banana, frosted cornflakes, and 8 ounces of hot chocolate
3. Bacon, eggs, biscuits with butter, and 4 ounces orange juice
4. Toast, jelly, oatmeal with cream and sugar, and 4 ounces apple juice

37. Three hours after birth, a neonate born to a diabetic mother seems jittery, has a weak, high pitched cry, and has irregular respirations. The nurse notes that these signs are often associated with:
1. Hypervolemia
2. Hypoglycemia
3. Hypocalcemia
4. Hyperglycemia

38. A newborn has Down syndrome. The mother says the cause of the abnormality was probably a viral infection she had in the fourth month of her pregnancy. The nurse recognizes that:
1. This abnormality appears in the baby's first cells
2. The fourth month is the worst time to have a virus
3. Viral agents can cause chromosomal abnormalities
4. This condition stems from nutritional deficiencies early in pregnancy

39. When assessing disturbed children the clue that would be most indicative of severe emotional problems would be a child's:
1. Physical complaints
2. Behavioral outbursts
3. Poor school performance
4. Unresponsiveness to the environment

40. The nurse in the labor and delivery department is informed that the client is a multipara. This would establish that the client:
1. Has a twin gestation
2. Has two or more living children at home
3. Had a multiple birth with her last pregnancy
4. Has had two or more deliveries reaching viability

41. A young male client who has been flirtatious with several of the younger nurses gives a bead bracelet that he made in occupational therapy to one of them. The most therapeutic response by the nurse would be:
1. "Thank you, but I can't accept gifts."
2. "You want me to have this gift; why?"
3. "I think you should give this to your family."
4. "Wow, that's really nice, but hospital policy does not allow me to accept gifts."

42. A man who has had a long history of alcohol abuse gets help and maintains sobriety. He turns to religion and frequently preaches against the abuse of alcohol and drugs. This client is demonstrating the use of:
1. Denial
2. Projection
3. Intellectualization
4. Reaction formation

43. On the fourth day after coronary artery bypass surgery (CABG), a client complains of feeling very tired. The BP is 126/70, the apical heart rate is 72, potassium is 4.0 mEq/L, urine output is 160 mL for 4 hours. Arterial blood gases are pH 7.34, PCO_2 46, PO_2 86, HCO_3 22. The nurse should:
1. Encourage the client to drink fluids
2. Cough and deep breathe the client
3. Reassure the client that this is a normal feeling
4. Encourage the client to choose potassium-rich foods

44. A 50-year-old with dyspnea and a productive cough is diagnosed as having pneumonia. An antitussive agent is ordered by the physician. The nurse explains that the purpose of this medication is to:
1. Inhibit the cough reflex
2. Prevent bronchospasms
3. Liquefy pulmonary secretions
4. Reduce lung tissue inflammation

45. An elderly female client who was hospitalized with bacterial meningitis is to be discharged. The husband is very concerned and anxious about his wife and the diagnosis. The nurse's intervention should be primarily concerned with:
1. Assisting him to make rational decisions
2. Determining his priority needs for information
3. Identifying support personnel in the community
4. Minimizing his interactions with his wife until discharge

46. When preparing a nursing care plan for a client who has incurred an electrical burn, the nurse checks the most recent laboratory tests. The finding the nurse would expect to see is:
1. A hemodilution of venous blood indicating early fluid shifts
2. A shift to the right in the WBC, indicating increased immune system activity
3. A magnetic resonance image of the various depths of the burn injury surrounding the entrance and exit points
4. The presence of hyperkalemia and hyperuricemia as potassium and uric acid precursors are released from dead or damaged cells

47. An immediate plan of action for a client with severe depression should include:
1. Focusing on the client's feelings of fear
2. Changing the client's manipulative behavior
3. Avoiding discussion of unanswerable questions
4. Establishing adequate nutrition, hydration, and elimination

48. A 2-year-old is diagnosed as autistic. The nurse recognizes that the constellation of behaviors specific to this disorder would include:
1. Twirling behavior, hallucinations, and delusions
2. Clinging, self-destructive behavior, and rudimentary attempts to communicate

3. Preoccupation with objects, a personal language, and various self-stimulating behaviors
4. Superior intellectual development, resistance to change, and a need for eye contact with adults

49. The two most common anxiety disorders in children are:
1. Phobias and sleep disturbances
2. Autism and childhood schizophrenia
3. Hyperactivity and attention deficit disorder
4. Affective disorders and antisocial behavior

50. A 7-month-old infant admitted with diarrhea due to a viral infection is diagnosed as having sickle cell anemia. The comment by the mother that indicates a readiness to learn genetic information about this disorder would be:
1. "When will my infant get over this condition?"
2. "What does diarrhea have to do with abnormal blood?"
3. "Why is it that our other children are not sick with the disease?"
4. "Where can we go to get the truth about why our infant is sick?"

51. To meet a hospitalized toddler's developmental needs it would be most appropriate for the nurse to:
1. Give the child several choices
2. Involve the parents in the child's care
3. Describe procedures in detail to the child
4. Place the child with a roommate of the same age

52. A client at 35 weeks' gestation is admitted to the obstetrical unit with painless uterine bleeding and a soft fundus. The nurse suspects:
1. Prolapsed cord
2. Placenta previa
3. Abruptio placentae
4. Disseminated intravascular coagulopathy

53. Most cesarean deliveries are performed primarily:
1. To prevent legal suits
2. As a repeat procedure
3. For the safety of the fetus
4. To ensure the safety of the mother

54. Evidence that a new mother has understood the instructions on caring for her son's circumcision would be found in the statement, "I need to:
1. Remove the yellow pus."
2. Pull back the remaining foreskin daily."
3. Keep the bandage on for the next week."
4. Wash my son's penis gently with warm water."

55. A 6-year-old is admitted with a diagnosis of acute glomerulonephritis. The nurse assesses the child for:
1. Cystitis
2. Hematuria
3. Hypothermia
4. Generalized edema

56. A 16-year-old with diabetes mellitus develops diabetic ketoacidosis. The nurse realizes that this condition can be caused by:
1. Skipping a meal
2. Eating a candy bar
3. Taking too little insulin
4. Increasing daily exercise

57. A client has sustained a head injury in an accident. The client is not oriented to time or place and must be called loudly several times to elicit a response. The client states both given name and surname with difficulty and cannot remember the accident. The nursing diagnosis requiring immediate intervention at this time is:
1. Fluid volume deficit
2. Ineffective airway clearance
3. Sensory/perceptual alterations
4. Altered cerebral tissue perfusion

58. A client with 70% of the body surface area burned has been evaluated for fluid requirements. A fluid resuscitation regimen using physiologic (0.9%) sodium chloride is started and the client develops generalized tissue edema and pulmonary edema. The nurse would expect the physician to:
1. Stop the fluid resuscitation and give diuretics
2. Order a more dilute form of fluid resuscitation
3. Convert to an IV fluid with a higher osmolarity
4. Establish a temporary line for emergency hemodialysis

59. A client admitted for a laser cholecystectomy is concerned about the postoperative recovery period. The nurse begins preoperative teaching by stating, "You will:
1. Be in the hospital for 3 or 4 days."
2. Have 3 or 4 one inch abdominal incisions."
3. Have a large abdominal incision and dressing."
4. Have a patient controlled analgesia (PCA) system for pain relief."

60. An important goal of nursing care for a client following coronary artery bypass surgery would be:
1. Increasing fluid intake
2. Beginning discharge planning
3. Encouraging activity and range of motion
4. Identifying cardiopulmonary complications

61. A client delivers an appropriate-for-gestational-age baby at 4:30 AM by vaginal delivery. At 9:00 AM the nurse notes that the client's fundus is firm and one finger above and deviated to the right of the umbilicus, the lochia is moderate rubra, and the urinary output has been 200 mL since delivery. The nurse's first action should be to:
1. Catheterize the client
2. Take the client's vital signs
3. Palpate the client's bladder
4. Massage the client's fundus

62. A young client is diagnosed as having Hodgkin's disease. The nursing care for this client should include:
1. Reassuring the client that a normal life-style can be maintained
2. Recognizing the grieving process and the need for the client to express it
3. Limiting the discussion of the diagnosis to reduce the occurrence of depression
4. Focusing on the positive aspects of life and encouragement to continue all activities

63. A client with closed head trauma undergoes placement of an intraventricular catheter and is being observed postsurgically. The nurse notes the client has become less alert and more difficult to arouse. The systolic blood pressure is increasing while the diastolic pressure is remaining stable. The client's heart and respiratory rates are decreasing. It would be most important for the nurse to:
1. Increase elevation of the client's position
2. Apply light suction to the drainage catheter

3. Notify the physician of the findings immediately
4. Engage the client in activity such as deep breathing

64. When evaluating the client with AIDS who has an absolute cell count of 500 mm^3 CD_4 cells and is receiving zidovudine (Retrovir), the nurse should observe for:
1. An intense renal toxicity
2. A decrease in CD_4 cells
3. A decrease in red blood cells
4. An increase in the hemoglobin

65. A client is admitted with atrial fibrillation, chronic peripheral edema, subnormal cardiac output, oliguria, and poor response to digitalis. A permanent pacemaker is inserted. The nurse recognizes that the pacemaker placement was successful when the client exhibits:
1. A weight gain
2. Increased urine output
3. A slower respiratory rate
4. Normal serum electrolytes

66. The nurse is aware that long-term chronic lung disease, such as cystic fibrosis, manifests itself in children by:
1. Inspiratory stridor
2. Hypertrophy of tonsils
3. Recurrent otitis media
4. Barrel shape to the chest

67. A child is found wandering in the park and is brought to the pediatric unit. The child weighs 27 pounds and is 30 inches tall, runs with a wide based stance, has a vocabulary of 500 words, has 20 deciduous teeth, and is shy with strangers. Based on the data collected, the nurse assesses that the child's age is:
1. 15 months
2. 24 months
3. 30 months
4. 40 months

68. A play activity that would be most effective in preventing pneumonia in the toddler with AIDS would be:
1. Fingerpainting
2. Reading a story
3. Blowing bubbles
4. Building with blocks

69. A 16-year-old primigravida is admitted with a diagnosis of mild preeclampsia. The nurse should notify the client's physician that her condition is worsening when the client becomes hyperreflexic, complains of epigastric discomfort, or develops:
   1. Fever
   2. Oliguria
   3. Thrombi
   4. Hypotension

70. A client's preterm labor is successfully suppressed. As part of the discharge plan, the nurse, to prevent further preterm labor, should teach the client to:
   1. Avoid breast stimulation and sexual activity
   2. Maintain her fluid intake at 1500 mL per day
   3. Focus on the date she is expected to deliver
   4. Remain on strict bedrest in the left lateral position

71. Immediately after a liver biopsy, a client is placed on the right side. The nurse tells the client that this position should be maintained for 60 to 90 minutes because it will:
   1. Help stop bleeding if any occurs
   2. Restore circulating blood volume
   3. Be the position of greatest comfort
   4. Help reduce fluid trapped in the biliary ducts

72. As a client enters the emergency department on a stretcher following an automobile accident the client asks the nurse, "Am I going to be alright?" The statement by the nurse that would be most therapeutic would be:
   1. "Tell me about your pain."
   2. "Yes, you've made it this far. You'll be okay."
   3. "I'm going to begin taking care of you right away."
   4. "Try to remain calm. You need to conserve your strength."

73. A client with human immunodeficiency virus (HIV) has diarrhea. It would be most therapeutic to teach the client to avoid:
   1. Potassium-rich food
   2. Raw fruits and vegetables
   3. Canned and frozen products
   4. Liquid nutritional supplements

74. A client with congestive heart failure has been on furosemide (Lasix) for several months. The comment made by the client that would indicate a side effect of the drug is:
   1. "I feel so weak and I have diarrhea frequently."
   2. "Even though I'm drinking lots of water, I still feel thirsty."
   3. "My legs feel weak and my heart is doing flip flops in my chest."
   4. "I'm having trouble getting my breath, even though I try to breathe deeply."

75. A client with a cancerous lesion of the bladder is to be treated with intravesicular thiotepa. Preoperatively, the nurse should explain that, prior to infusion of the thiotepa into the bladder, the client should expect:
   1. Instillation of BCG vaccine
   2. Partial excision of the bladder
   3. Removal of organs surrounding the bladder
   4. Electrical cauterization of the cancerous tissue

Comprehensive examination 2

76. An 11-year-old talks to the school nurse about an episode of disruptive, acting-out behavior. The child states, "I had a stomach ache and felt like vomiting. I couldn't help it. I was just so mad at my dad." The nurse's most appropriate response would be:
    1. "I can see that you are angry. Let's look at better ways to express it."
    2. "Perhaps it would be helpful if you let your dad know that you are angry."
    3. "If you can get rid of your anger, perhaps your stomach ache will go away."
    4. "I can understand your anger, but you can't continue to disrupt the classroom."

77. A 4-year-old with leukemia comes to the clinic for chemotherapy. All of the blood work is normal except for a platelet count of 30,000 mm (30 x 103/mm^3). The nursing diagnosis that would address this problem would be:
    1. Fatigue related to effects of elevated platelet count
    2. High risk for injury: infection related to low platelet count
    3. High risk for injury: bleeding related to low platelet count
    4. Altered nutrition: less than body requirements related to elevated platelet count

78. Assessment of an 8-year-old child newly casted in the emergency department following fracture of the left tibia should include monitoring:
    1. Muscular status
    2. Respiratory status
    3. Neurovascular status
    4. Socioeconomic status

79. Anxiety can best be described as:
    1. An experience that results from a loss of self-esteem
    2. A feeling of uneasiness that warns against involvement
    3. A common reaction emerging from the use of defense mechanisms
    4. A vague, uneasy feeling that occurs when the self-concept is threatened

80. The nurse evaluates that a new mother may not be bonding with her newborn when she:
    1. Unwraps the baby then uses only her fingertips to explore for all the body parts
    2. Comments that the baby seems to settle down when the baby starts to thumb suck
    3. Takes the baby from the nurse and holds the baby at arms length to make eye contact
    4. Calls the nurse to take her baby back to the nursery and change the diaper because it is soiled

81. An infant has just returned to the unit after a cardiac catheterization. It would be most important for the nurse to monitor for:
    1. A fluid and electrolyte deficit related to surgery
    2. Hemorrhage related to femoral artery operative site
    3. An alteration in cardiac output related to cardiac defect
    4. Any cardiac dysrhythmia related to cardiac catheterization

82. For rigid clubfoot deformities, treatment should be initiated in the first week after birth. The nurse is aware that the primary reason for immediate treatment is that:
    1. Early treatment helps to allay parents' anxiety
    2. Casting is only effective immediately after birth
    3. Complications of treatment are less severe early after birth
    4. Soft tissue changes become more rigid if treatment is delayed

83. A 3-year-old is brought to the emergency room with a high fever, 104° F (40° C), a muffled voice, drooling, and severe respiratory retractions. The nurse's first priority should be to:
    1. Notify the physician immediately
    2. Administer an antipyretic for the fever
    3. Give the child oral liquids to help reduce the fever
    4. Place the child in an upright position and provide oxygen

84. When preparing the discharge teaching plan for a client following an aortic bypass, the nurse should emphasize instructions relative to:
    1. Digoxin (Lanoxin)
    2. Heparin sodium (Heparin)
    3. Warfarin sodium (Coumadin)
    4. Vitamin K (AquaMEPHYTON)

85. A client with severe abdominal pain begins vomiting a brown, fecal-smelling emesis. Before notifying the physician, it would be most important for the nurse to:
    1. Auscultate the client's abdomen for bowel sounds

32

2. Insert a nasogastric tube and apply it to intermittent suction
3. Perform a digital rectal exam inspecting for fecal impaction
4. Submit a sample of the emesis to the lab for occult blood analysis

86. A client with edema has been evaluated for congestive heart failure, renal failure, and liver dysfunction; each condition has been ruled out as a cause of the edema. During interdisciplinary rounds, the client's team is discussing interventions that would focus on the etiology. Toward this goal, it would be most insightful for the nursing care coordinator to recommend:
1. Placing the client on diuretics
2. Obtaining a nutritional evaluation
3. Increasing the client's daily activity
4. Monitoring the client's urine output

87. Discharge instructions to a breastfeeding mother of a newborn who has physiologic jaundice would include that the mother report if her baby:
1. Becomes reluctant to breastfeed
2. Begins having loose yellow stools
3. Begins waking every 2 to 3 hours
4. Frequently passes pale yellow urine

88. Following a cesarean delivery a client develops disseminated intravascular coagulation (DIC). The nurse prepares the client for transfer to the:
1. Coronary care unit for close observation
2. Nursing unit for routine postpartum observations
3. Operating room for a total abdominal hysterectomy
4. Surgical intensive care unit for hemodynamic monitoring

89. A client has had an uneventful pregnancy until labor begins. The client is admitted with a painful, rigid abdomen and ultrasound reveals a large amount of blood concealed in the uterus. The nurse suspects:
1. Placenta previa
2. Ectopic pregnancy
3. Abruptio placentae
4. Incomplete abortion

90. A client with Graves' disease should be monitored for thyroid storm or thyrotoxic crisis. The nurse should notify the physician if the client has:
1. Extra-dry skin
2. Dyspnea on exertion

3. A pulse of 95 beats per minute
4. A temperature of 100.8°F (38.22°C)

91. A client is to receive meperidine (Demerol) 75 mg and hydroxyzine (Vistaril) 25 mg IM. Available is meperidine 100 mg per 2 mL and hydroxyzine 50 mg per 1 mL. When the dosage is drawn up in a single syringe, the nurse should administer:
1. 1.25 mL
2. 1.5 mL
3. 1.75 mL
4. 2 mL

92. A 27-year-old male is admitted to a psychiatric unit on a temporary detention order. The nurse finds the client staring out of a window with his eyes rapidly scanning the cars six floors below. The client appears to be responding to voices and continually attempts to open the window lock. The client does not respond when called by name. The nurse should assess:
1. What the voices are saying to the client
2. A description of what the client sees out of the window
3. Whether the client is thinking about jumping out of the window
4. The extent of the client's knowledge about window lock operation

93. The nurse should encourage the parents of a child who is autistic to emphasize:
1. Maintaining structure in the child's daily activities
2. Playing the television or radio constantly as a distraction, or stimulus
3. Using physical touch as much as possible to hold the child's attention
4. Speaking in descriptive sentences to enhance the child's language development

94. The condition of a client with advanced chronic obstructive pulmonary disease (COPD) is deteriorating. The nurse should notify the physician immediately if the client develops a:
1. PaO_2 of 38 mmHg
2. Tidal volume of 750
3. $PaCO_2$ of 65 mmHg
4. Respiratory rate of 28

33

95. A 65-year-old client with deep vein thrombophlebitis is receiving intravenous heparin and develops numbness of the lower extremities. The physician is notified immediately and orders coagulation studies. The nurse should also expect the physician to:
   1. Order a stat MRI of the spine
   2. Evaluate the client for hypokalemia
   3. Stop the heparin infusion immediately
   4. Instruct the nurse to give protamine sulfate

96. A 60-year-old client comes to the diabetic clinic. Noninsulin-dependent diabetes mellitus is suspected. When obtaining a nursing history the nurse would expect this older client to indicate:
   1. A rapid onset of symptoms
   2. A recent episode of ketosis
   3. A "sweet tooth" but no obesity
   4. An insidious onset with fatigue

97. A 4-year-old is admitted for a cardiac catheterization. The nurse is aware that the statement by the mother that should be brought to the attention of the admitting physician is, "My child:
   1. Is short of breath after playing vigorously."
   2. Has been upset and crying all during the trip to the hospital."
   3. Has sisters who have been home with the flu for the past week."
   4. Doesn't seem to be growing at the same rate as her classmates."

98. Based on knowledge of growth and development, the nurse should recognize that the optimal time for repair of epispadias is:
   1. Just before puberty
   2. After the child begins school
   3. Between 3 and 5 years of age
   4. Between 6 and 18 months of age

99. A child with an HIV infection is receiving didanosine (ddi). The response that indicates the development of an adverse reaction to this drug would be the development of:
   1. Muscle wasting
   2. Growth retardation
   3. A learning disability
   4. Peripheral neuropathy

100. The nurse observes that a client with a newly placed tracheostomy tube that has a removable inner cannula is becoming restless. When auscultating the lungs, the nurse notes normal breath sounds on the left and decreased breath sounds on the right. The most appropriate initial response from the nurse would be to:
   1. Remove and clean the inner cannula of the tracheostomy tube
   2. Flush the tracheostomy with sterile saline and suction the client
   3. Administer supplemental oxygen to the client via the tracheostomy collar
   4. Oxygenate the client using a manual resuscitator bag and suction the tracheostomy

101. The physician tells the nurse that a client's aortic aneurysm is extending. The signs or symptoms that the nurse would expect to observe are:
   1. Increased abdominal and back pain
   2. Decreased pulse rate and palpitations
   3. Retrosternal chest pain radiating to left arm
   4. Elevated blood pressure and rapid respirations

102. Following maxillofacial trauma, a client requires intermaxillary fixation with interdental wiring. The client vomits postsurgically and is unable to expectorate the emesis. The nurse should:
   1. Attempt to suction the emesis from the client's mouth and throat by nasal and/or oral suctioning
   2. Quickly install a nasogastric tube suctioning the airway as the tube is being passed by the pharynx
   3. Immediately cut the interdental wiring allowing the client to open the mouth and eliminate the emesis
   4. Sit the client up in a forward-leaning position and instruct the client to force the emesis out of the spaces behind the molars

103. During the early postoperative period following a colectomy, a nurse suspects a client is bleeding internally. The client is assessed for changes in the vital signs. The findings that would most support the nurse's suspicion would be:
   1. Increased blood pressure and apical heart rate
   2. Decreased blood pressure and apical heart rate
   3. Increased blood pressure and decreased apical heart rate
   4. Decreased blood pressure and increased apical heart rate

104. A client who had experienced an episode of preterm labor that was treated with tocolytic medications is to be discharged. The nurse evaluates that there is a good understanding of the teaching regarding the prevention of another episode when the client states:
    1. "I know I have to just take one day at a time."
    2. "I never drink anything except with my meals."
    3. "We have a nice comfortable couch in the lounge at work."
    4. "My husband and I have always enjoyed just being together."

105. A client who had an abruptio placentae is now one day postpartum. The nurse assesses petechiae on the client's abdomen and a large bruise on the upper arm. The nurse should:
    1. Start an IV of normal saline
    2. Report this to the physician
    3. Order appropriate laboratory work
    4. Do nothing because this is normal

106. A client who is taking tamoxifen (Nolvadex) for cancer of the breast tells the nurse she is nauseous, feels tired, and has no appetite. She also states that she urinates more often at night than she wants to. The nurse should:
    1. Further assess the client for signs of clinical depression
    2. Ask the family if the client is taking more pain medication than she should
    3. Assess the client for fluid and electrolyte imbalance, especially hypercalcemia
    4. Inform the physician that the client is demonstrating toxic side effects of tamoxifen

107. A 34-year-old, male client, on the progressive coronary care unit has been making statements of grandiosity such as, "I really know more than any of you nurses and doctors combined!" Furthermore, the nurse suspects the client has been noncompliant and neglectful with medications and self-care. This should lead the nurse to recognize that the client has:
    1. High level anxiety
    2. Feelings of hopelessness
    3. A body-image disturbance
    4. A disturbance in self-esteem

108. An example of a secondary prevention activity that the mental health nurse performs in an outpatient setting would be:
    1. Organizing community action groups to plan for legislative changes
    2. Monitoring a client's adjustment after discharge from an inpatient unit
    3. Conducting a resocialization group for clients with chronic schizophrenia
    4. Referring clients for inpatient treatment based upon a mental status examination

109. The basic therapeutic tool of the psychiatric/mental health nurse is:
    1. The self
    2. Group discussion
    3. A knowledge base
    4. An ability to disclose

110. Immediately following a bilateral adrenalectomy, a client is receiving dextrose 5% in normal saline at a rate of 300 mL per hour intravenously. The nurse should know to contact the physician if the:
    1. Client's hourly urine output exceeds 200 milliliters
    2. Client develops jugular vein distention and orthopnea
    3. Client's urine specific gravity and osmolarity decrease
    4. Client experiences pain at the site of the intravenous insertion

111. Following a minor automobile accident and arrest for DWI, a client with a long history of alcohol abuse is brought to the emergency service. The client is pacing and appears confused, malnourished, and extremely dehydrated. After admission the priority nursing diagnosis for this client would be:
    1. Agitation related to fears
    2. Sleep pattern disturbance related to restlessness
    3. Risk for injury related to environmental misperceptions
    4. Risk for fluid volume deficit related to altered intake and loss

112. Following abdominal surgery, a client's urine output decreases to 15 mL/hr for 2 consecutive hours. The nurse should:
    1. Change the catheter
    2. Notify the physician
    3. Increase the IV rate
    4. Monitor the output for another hour

113. When planning to alleviate a client's anxiety about pulmonary surgery, the nurse would consider that the anxiety may be reduced if the client is:
    1. Willing to communicate concerns
    2. Oriented to time, place, and person
    3. Correctly outlining the treatment plan
    4. Able to verbalize increased self-esteem

114. It is important for the nurse teaching a client with hyperthyroidism to encourage the client to:
    1. Increase the nutritional intake
    2. Maintain a warm ambient temperature
    3. Institute regular but reduced hours of sleep
    4. Develop a regimen of gradually increased activity

115. A client with chronic obstructive pulmonary disease is receiving theophylline (Theo-Dur). When teaching the client about the side effects of this drug it is most important for the nurse to include:
    1. Anorexia
    2. Palpitations
    3. Drowsiness
    4. Constipation

116. When assessing a client diagnosed with multiple personality disorder, who has been experiencing fugue states, the nurse would expect to identify:
    1. No history of psychiatric problems
    2. A strong creative and artistic ability
    3. Poor comprehension and intellectual capacity
    4. A difficulty in remembering concurrent experiences

117. At 2 months of age an infant returns for surgical repair of a cleft lip. Preoperatively the child is fitted for a (an):
    1. Vest restraint
    2. Wrist restraint
    3. Elbow restraint
    4. Mummy restraint

118. A male client complains that he is unable to void after a cystoscopy. The nurse should:
    1. Limit oral fluids until he voids
    2. Assure him that this is normal
    3. Insert a urinary retention catheter
    4. Palpate above the pubic symphysis

119. Fetal anomalies are detected by amniocentesis through the examination of fetal:

    1. Blood chemistry
    2. Excretions in the fluid
    3. Cells sloughed into the fluid
    4. L/S (lecithin/sphingomyelin) ratio

120. The nurse recognizes that a pregnant multipara has understood the relationship of prostaglandin gel to cervical ripening prior to induction when the client:
    1. Tells her children she will be home in a few hours
    2. States she is glad that this labor will be shorter than her others
    3. Tells her family that they will have a new member by the next day
    4. States she has made arrangements for child care for the next several days

121. One of the most effective means for the nurse to prevent neonatal hypoglycemia is to encourage:
    1. A first feeding of 10% glucose water
    2. Glucose water 5% after breastfeeding
    3. Early frequent breastfeeding after birth
    4. Supplemental formula with the breastfeeding

122. The nurse is aware that the coping mechanism of denial is frequently used by families of children with acyanotic heart disease because:
    1. Acyanotic heart disease often results from a genetic defect
    2. Children with acyanotic heart disease are less likely to be symptomatic
    3. Cyanosis only develops after extensive exertion in acyanotic heart disease
    4. Surgery tends to be delayed in children who are acyanotic, causing more anxiety

123. A client with pregnancy-induced hypertension is admitted to the hospital in early labor and placed on magnesium sulfate. The nurse should:
    1. Test the knee jerk reflex and administer the medication only if the reflexes are present
    2. Check the urinary output and continue the medication if it is less than 100 mL every 4 hr
    3. Count the respirations and continue the medication only if respirations are below 12 per minute
    4. Monitor for rapid progression of labor and decrease the oxytocin flow rate before administering the medication

124. The nurse in the prenatal clinic is offering a sibling preparation education class. The primary purpose of this class is to:

1. Help the children understand infant safety
2. Acquaint the children with the birth process
3. Assist the children to feel part of the family
4. Teach the children how they can help the mother

125. A priority intervention for a client in the manic phase of a bipolar disorder would be to:
    1. Increase the client's feelings of self-worth
    2. Promote the client's leisure and social skills
    3. Emphasize the client's ability to express feelings
    4. Establish rapport and build a trusting relationship

126. A public health nurse is asked to speak to a group of individuals about acquired immune deficiency syndrome (AIDS). When identifying individuals at high risk for developing AIDS, the nurse states:
    1. "Children with hemophilia have a 40% chance of contracting AIDS."
    2. "Unmarried, sexually active women have the highest incidence of AIDS."
    3. "The people at greatest risk for contracting AIDS are those who use cocaine."
    4. "Over 50% of new AIDS cases are in men who have had both homosexual and bisexual relations."

127. A 28-year-old female is transferred to the medical floor 1 week after admission for a spinal cord injury at L5 after a motor vehicle accident. The client's history shows that consciousness was not lost, there is full function of the arms, and flaccidity is present in both legs. To prevent complications from bed rest, the nurse should give priority to:
    1. Setting up an overhead trapeze
    2. Checking both legs for evidence of pressure
    3. Maintaining the foot of the bed in dependent position
    4. Placing the head of the bed in the high-Fowler's position

128. An infant weighs 6 lbs (2722 g) at delivery. At 12 months of age the infant is brought to the well baby clinic for a checkup. The finding that indicates the goal of promoting normal growth and development has been met is, "The infant:
    1. Weighs 19 lb (8618 g)."
    2. Sits up with some assistance."
    3. Exhibits a positive Moro reflex."
    4. Has a vocabulary of 10 to 20 words."

129. Postoperatively, after closure of a myelomeningocele sac, the nurse plans infant positioning. The position that is optimal for preventing hip dislocation is:
    1. Supine with knees flexed
    2. Side-lying, either right or left
    3. Semi-Fowler's in an infant seat
    4. Prone with hips and legs abducted

130. A 9-year-old is referred to the school nurse by the teacher because of hostile, acting-out behavior. The child has also complained of nausea and abdominal cramping. The nurse assesses the cause of this behavior when the child states:
    1. "My older sister is having stomach aches and headaches too."
    2. "My mother works and I don't like to worry her with my stomach aches."
    3. "I ate only a little cereal and drank a glass of orange juice this morning."
    4. "My dad isn't coming home any more and I don't like what's happening."

131. An 8-year-old with an attention-deficit/hyperactivity disorder is jumping off the hospital bed onto a chair. Initially the nurse can most effectively handle this situation by stating:
    1. "I need to talk to you."
    2. "Stop that, this instant!"
    3. "You are going to hurt yourself."
    4. "Why would you do something like that?"

132. A client with acute schizophrenia refuses to eat telling the nurse, "I do not like the food in the hospital because it has chemicals that electrify me." Initially the nurse should:
    1. Allow the client to order meals from a local restaurant
    2. Have a family member bring food during visiting hours
    3. Provide foods for the client that are served in closed containers
    4. Provide finger food so the client can eat alone while walking around

133. The most prohibiting factor for use of the antipsychotic medication clozapine (Clozaril) is:
    1. Most clients refuse to take the drug
    2. That it has not proven very effective
    3. That it causes severe blood dyscrasias
    4. Inconvenience because blood tests must be done weekly

134. Soon after undergoing a fasciotomy of the left leg, a client attempts to sit on the edge of the bed with the feet on the floor. The client rapidly becomes syncopic and falls. Upon finding the client on the floor, the nurse's initial response should be to:
 1. Get help returning the client to bed
 2. Establish the client's responsiveness
 3. Ensure the client's left leg is elevated
 4. Assess the client for associated injuries

135. A client with a history of 36 hours of frequent diarrheal stools is seen in the emergency department. The client has been compensating for the diarrhea by drinking large amounts of water. An electrolyte panel is drawn: the serum sodium is 130 mEq/L and the glucose is 180 mg/dL. If fluid is administered in the emergency department, the nurse should expect it to be:
 1. Saline 0.9%
 2. Saline 0.45%
 3. Dextrose 5% in water
 4. Dextrose 5% in 0.45% saline

136. A 70-year-old client comes to the clinic for care of pyrosis (heartburn). This symptom is worse after eating and at night. The instruction by the nurse that might be most helpful is:
 1. Avoid nonfat milk in the diet
 2. Lie on the right side when sleeping
 3. Limit the coffee and chocolate consumed
 4. Assume the Trendelenburg position when lying down

137. A male client appears to be having a dystonic reaction to his tranquilizer. His head is twisted to one side, and he cannot straighten his neck. The nurse is aware that the medications commonly used to treat dystonias include:
 1. Mellaril, Prolixin, Trilafon
 2. Haldol, Navane, Thorazine
 3. Artane, Benadryl, Cogentin
 4. Stelazine, Prozac, Phenergan

138. During the first 24 hours after a bilateral adrenalectomy, a client is receiving intravenous cortisol. The nurse caring for the client should expect to routinely monitor capillary glucose levels because:
 1. Stress from surgery lowers serum glucose levels
 2. A side effect of cortisol therapy is hyperglycemia

3. Removal of an adrenal gland often leads to hyperglycemia
 4. Cortisol therapy depresses gluconeogenesis and lowers blood sugar

139. The husband of a 23-year-old client who is 3 weeks postpartum tells the nurse in the clinic, "My wife has not been eating or sleeping and has not been caring for herself or our baby." The wife, who had been employed as a nursery school teacher, makes no eye contact with the nurse and when spoken to gives no answer or responds with one or two words. A possible nursing diagnosis for this client would be:
 1. Anxiety related to change in role functioning
 2. Impaired adjustment related to assault on self-esteem
 3. Ineffective family coping related to family disorganization and role changes
 4. Altered role performance related to change in usual patterns or responsibility

140. A 36-year-old primigravida whose pregnancy has been unremarkable arrives for a regular prenatal visit at 34 weeks gestation. Her only complaint is slight puffiness in her hands and ankles. The nurse becomes concerned when assessment of the client reveals:
 1. An increase in fetal activity
 2. A blood pressure of 140/88
 3. A serum glucose of 120 mg/dL
 4. A loss of 1 pound since the last visit

141. A 12-hour-old neonate begins manifesting cyanosis, hypothermia, lethargy, and feeding problems. The nurse should assess the baby's blood:
 1. Calcium level
 2. Glucose level
 3. Bilirubin level
 4. Magnesium level

142. The nurse teaches the mother of a child with congenital aganglionic megacolon (Hirschsprung disease) to administer:
 1. Tap water enemas
 2. Soapsuds enemas
 3. Phosphate enemas
 4. Normal saline enemas

143. A client is admitted to the emergency unit with multiple old and new tracking scars indicating drug abuse. When performing the admission assessment the nurse should expect the client to reveal a history of:
   1. Inadequate financial resources
   2. Taking a variety of drugs simultaneously
   3. Long periods of psychosocial depression
   4. Loneliness or isolation from family members

144. A maturational crisis differs from a situational crisis because of its:
   1. Severity
   2. Duration
   3. Outcome
   4. Predictability

145. After making the nursing diagnosis of impaired verbal communication related to psychologic barriers, it would be most therapeutic for the nurse to:
   1. Involve the client's family in self-care activities
   2. Invite the client to view sports on TV with the staff
   3. Establish and maintain a daily routine for the client
   4. Spend time with the client even if the client does not respond

146. When assessing for the development of an infection following the application of a plaster cast to the leg, the nurse should teach the client to observe for the presence of:
   1. Hot spots
   2. Cold toes
   3. Warm toes
   4. Paresthesia

147. In preparation for hemodialysis, a client with kidney failure undergoes placement of an arteriovenous fistula in the right arm. To help prevent postsurgical complications, the nurse should instruct the client to:
   1. Avoid lying or sleeping on the right side
   2. Attempt to maintain the right arm in flexion
   3. Wear a firm gauze wrap over the site to prevent bleeding
   4. Refrain from exercises that involve use of the right hand

148. Four hours after a head injury, the client's pulse pressure is increasing and respirations are very slow and irregular. The client no longer responds to verbal stimulation. Arterial blood gases drawn immediately reveal: PCO_2 48, pH 7.33, HCO_3 22. The nurse is aware that the physician's order, which has the highest priority, is:
   1. Orally intubate and place on ventilator
   2. Give mannitol intravenous bolus over 30 minutes
   3. Insert subarachnoid intracranial pressure monitor
   4. Administer dexamethasone sodium phosphate IV push

149. The nurse plans to use a high-Fowler's position for a client who is experiencing:
   1. Orthopnea
   2. A pleural friction rub
   3. A nonproductive cough
   4. Oxygen supplementation

150. To prevent tissue inflammation associated with the parenteral administration of phenytoin (Dilantin) the nurse should:
   1. Apply ice to the IM puncture site
   2. Use a large vein for IV administration
   3. Check the administration site twice a day
   4. Keep the drug refrigerated prior to administration

Comprehensive examination 3

151. The nursing action that is most appropriate when considering the psychologic aspect of elective termination of a pregnancy is:
    1. Allowing the client to grieve her loss
    2. Being quiet and saying little to the client
    3. Explaining the steps in the abortion process
    4. Telling the client all that is happening but not discussing the pregnancy

152. A client has a cardiac catheterization and returns to the unit. When evaluating the effects of the catheterization, the nurse checks the apical pulse for one full minute because:
    1. Lanoxin is given routinely after cardiac catheterization
    2. Peripheral pulses are weaker after the catheterization procedure
    3. Vessel spasms can occur postcatheterization at the catheter site
    4. Cardiac dysrhythmia is a possible complication following catheterization

153. Staphylococcus aureus is growing in a leg ulcer of a client who has insulin-dependent diabetes mellitus. Because of this organism this client requires:
    1. Isolation
    2. Amputation
    3. Alcohol scrubs
    4. An acid-ash diet

154. A young man who sustained an open fracture of the right femur had an open reduction and internal fixation of the fracture and is now in balanced skeletal traction. The nurse recognizes that this:
    1. Keeps the femoral bone in alignment
    2. Permits the femoral bone to be mobile
    3. Improves circulation of the affected limb
    4. Increases mobilization until the fracture heals

155. A child with a fused cranium undergoes surgery for placement of a ventriculoperitoneal (VP) shunt. The goal that would be of highest priority when the child returns to the nursing unit is that:
    1. The child's shunt will remain patent as evidenced by an absence of vomiting, holding of the head, or irritability
    2. The child will remain free of infection as evidenced by no signs of incisional swelling or drainage, irritability, or lethargy

    3. The parents will be able to describe hydrocephalus and verbalize the necessity of shunt placement and the usual operative routine
    4. The child will be in fluid balance as evidenced by stable weight, good skin turgor, stable electrolytes, and moist mucous membranes

156. An 18-month-old has a repair of a cleft palate. Postoperatively the nurse recognizes that it would be most appropriate to give this baby fluids by use of a:
    1. Cup
    2. Straw
    3. Soft nipple
    4. Nasogastric tube

157. The appropriate response to a breastfeeding woman's concern over her neonate receiving adequate amounts of nutrients is:
    1. "You have a big strong baby who will let you know if there is not enough milk."
    2. "By nursing the baby right after birth and then every 2 to 3 hours, you will probably provide all that is needed."
    3. "We will begin supplemental feedings right away so you will not have to worry about there being enough milk."
    4. "If your baby starts losing weight, we can supplement the breastfeedings with formula until you have enough milk."

158. A pregnant client is diagnosed with deep vein thrombosis. The nurse prepares a solution of:
    1. Heparin calcium
    2. Warfarin sodium
    3. Protamine sulfate
    4. Coumadin sodium

159. Nursing assessment for the client with anorexia nervosa should focus on:
    1. Control issues
    2. Academic issues
    3. Peer relationships
    4. Family relationships

160. The mother of a 6-year-old boy with an attention-deficit/hyperactive disorder asks to speak to the nurse about her son's behavior. The nurse would be most therapeutic by saying, "Your son:
    1. Needs a firmer approach from you."
    2. Must be difficult to handle at home."
    3. Sure is active; he must wear you out."
    4. Is a cute child, but he needs to calm down."

161. As the nurse approaches a client with the diagnosis of major depression to begin a one-to-one relationship, the client states, "I don't think you should bother with me. I am not worthy of your attention." The most therapeutic statement by the nurse would be:
   1. "You sound so hopeless. Tell me what's on your mind."
   2. "I wouldn't be trying to help you if I didn't think you were worthy."
   3. "OK, I'll leave you alone for now, but I'll be back later to talk with you."
   4. "You are really down on yourself and that just makes things worse. Cheer up."

162. A client is admitted with a drug overdose. The priority nursing action when planning care for this client would be to:
   1. Support respiratory function
   2. Promptly measure vital signs
   3. Initiate measures to clear the intoxicant
   4. Check the client's belongings for additional drugs

163. A client, who has learned to survive by using assault, robbery, or similar combative strategies, is injured while being arrested. The client's statement to the nurse on the prison unit that indicates there may be a change in this antisocial attitude would be:
   1. "I have the right to survive."
   2. "I'm sorry I had to hit the old lady."
   3. "What's wrong with what I'm doing?"
   4. "Everyone takes something from somebody."

164. A client, who has been experiencing pain in the right calf for 2 days, notices that it is larger than the left. There is no past history of any medical problems. Upon examination, the right calf is edematous, warm, red, and tender to touch. As part of the assessment, the nurse should ask if the pain:
   1. Worsens in the morning upon arising
   2. Increases with activity and is alleviated with rest
   3. Is relieved by positioning the leg in a dependent position
   4. Is aggravated when the toes are pointed toward the knee

165. A client who has had pelvic surgery complains to the nurse of substernal chest pain and difficulty breathing. The client is diaphoretic, pale, and anxious. The first action by the nurse should be to:
   1. Call the physician
   2. Listen to breath sounds
   3. Check the blood pressure
   4. Raise the head of the bed

166. A client has been hospitalized with a heparin drip because of a pulmonary embolus. Once discharged, the client is to be maintained on Coumadin. The nurse's plan for discharge teaching should focus on:
   1. Incisional care
   2. Prevention of trauma
   3. Discussion of a high potassium diet
   4. Prevention of upper respiratory infections

167. A 7-year-old begins crutch-walking with assistance. The nursing intervention that will best help prevent injury to the child if a fall is considered inevitable is:
   1. Putting a safety helmet on the child
   2. Developing a distance goal for the child
   3. Allowing the child to walk only on carpeted floors
   4. Clearing the hallways prior to the child's ambulation

168. Before giving digoxin to a 3-month-old with tetralogy of Fallot, the nurse assesses the apical pulse and finds it is 110 beats per minute. The nurse should:
   1. Hold the drug because the heart rate is too low
   2. Notify the physician because the infant is having a toxic response to digoxin
   3. Notify the physician because tachycardia is an adverse response
   4. Administer the drug because this is a normal heart rate for a 3-month-old

169. A toddler is hospitalized after swallowing a penny. An X-ray reveals that the penny is lodged high in the esophagus. The most important nursing consideration when caring for this toddler is:
   1. Pushing fluids to promote movement of the penny
   2. Examining all stools to check for passage of the penny
   3. Keeping the child quiet to prevent aspiration of the penny
   4. Providing the child with age-appropriate diversional activities

170. A major goal for a female client recovering from a depression would be that the client:
    1. Contacts social services for assistance
    2. Interacts with her family and friends as before
    3. Verbalizes a willingness to change her life-style
    4. Requests an antidepressant medication be prescribed

171. A 16-year-old with a history of amphetamine abuse has just returned to the adolescent unit from a 4-hour pass. The nurse suspects that the adolescent may have taken amphetamines while on pass when assessment reveals:
    1. Retarded speech and immobility
    2. Hostile impulsiveness and irritability
    3. Constricted pupils with a blank stare
    4. Decreased pulse and blood pressure

172. The nursing assessments that would indicate adequate fluid resuscitation of a client who has had extensive full-thickness burns are:
    1. Polyuria and orthostatic hypotension
    2. Blood pressure of 130/80 and clear mentation
    3. Decreasing edema and CVP reading of 0 to 5 mmH$_2$O
    4. Urinary output of less than 30 mL/hr and increased pulse rate

173. A client's leg ulcer is being treated with twice-a-day povidone-iodine dressings and is showing no signs of new tissue growth. The nurse should expect the physician to:
    1. Leave the wound uncovered and open to air
    2. Debride the wound with wet-to-dry dressings
    3. Change to sterile normal saline for wound care
    4. Increase the frequency of the dressing changes

174. Total parenteral nutrition is a more desirable therapy than intravenous fluids for a client who is losing excessive weight. The nurse understands that, if a client were to receive only intravenous fluids, the weight loss would continue because of:
    1. The absence of bulk in the diet
    2. A decreased intake of carbohydrates
    3. An insufficient intake of fat-soluble vitamins
    4. The reduced concentration of electrolytes in IV fluid

175. The nurse is assessing a client with dementia. To effectively elicit information about the client's self-insight, the nurse should ask the client:
    1. "What does 4 + 4 − 2 equal?"
    2. "What do you think is wrong with you?"
    3. "What is the day and year of your birth?"
    4. "What is the name of the president of the United States?"

176. A depressed client has been taking fluoxetine (Prozac) for the past several weeks and has not demonstrated any improvement. The psychiatrist discontinues this drug and orders tranylcypromine sulfate (Parnate) 15 mg every 12 hours. The nurse should refuse to administer this medication because:
    1. The dosage is below that recommended by the drug manufacturer
    2. The dosage is higher that that recommended by the drug manufacturer
    3. First the dietician must educate the client about certain foods to prevent a hypertensive crisis
    4. It is contraindicated for clients who have taken other antidepressants such as fluoxetine (Prozac)

177. While caring for an infant with a cleft palate the nurse informs the parents that surgical correction is usually performed between 12 and 18 months of age, before the child:
    1. Acquires body image problems
    2. Evidences marked hearing loss
    3. Develops faulty speech patterns
    4. Falls behind in height and weight

178. A 10-year-old child, in traction for a fractured femur, has a nursing diagnosis of "Powerlessness." The nurse understands that the child would benefit most by:
    1. Developing a list of coping strategies
    2. Including family members in the care
    3. Visiting frequently with the peer group
    4. Providing as much self-care as possible

179. A 14-year-old is admitted with left testicular cancer. He is scheduled for removal of his left testicle. The nursing diagnosis with the highest priority preoperatively is:
    1. Anxiety related to threat to life
    2. Sexual dysfunction related to altered body structure

3. Body image disturbance related to biophysical changes
4. Knowledge deficit related to ignorance about testicular self-examination

180. A neonate who has been feeding well becomes lethargic, does not want to nurse, and has dark urine in the diaper. The nurse identifies that this neonate is exhibiting signs of:
1. Dehydration
2. Hypothermia
3. Hypoglycemia
4. Hyperbilirubinemia

181. After a client completes a chemotherapeutic regimen for cancer of the breast, tamoxifen (Nolvadex) is prescribed. The client states, "I understand that this medication is an extension of the chemotherapy. Do I still have cancer? Didn't they get all of it during surgery and the other chemotherapy?" The best reply by the nurse would be:
1. "Tamoxifen is an antiestrogen medication used to kill the cancer cells that remain."
2. "You know that cancer spreads so easily and it is impossible to get all the cells at one shot."
3. "What made you think of that idea? You know that between the surgery and the chemotherapy all of the cells should have been killed."
4. "Tamoxifen is an antiestrogen drug and, since your tumor responded to estrogen for growth, you are taking it to prevent recurrence."

182. A client in the thirty-eighth week of her first pregnancy is feeling fine, but the results of her weekly examination show a weight gain of five pounds, blood pressure of 144/92 and 1+ proteinuria. The client is hospitalized and placed on bedrest in a side lying position. The client asks the nurse why this is important. The nurse's response would be based on the knowledge that this position:
1. Decreases intraabdominal pressure
2. Lowers the blood pressure significantly
3. Moves edematous fluid to the extracellular space
4. Increases the circulation to the kidneys and uterus

183. A client, scheduled for continuous ambulatory peritoneal dialysis, asks the nurse what the procedure entails. The nurse's explanation includes information that:
1. Peritoneal dialysis is done in an ambulatory care clinic
2. There is continuous hemodialysis and peritoneal dialysis
3. About a quarter of a liter of dialysate is maintained intraperitoneally
4. There is continuous contact of dialysate with the peritoneal membrane

184. A client who is somewhat hostile and adamant about not having a blood pressure problem states that a recent physical revealed a blood pressure of 182/112. The client indicates that the doctor wants the blood pressure checked daily for 10 days. The client states this is too much of a bother. The nurse's best response would be:
1. "Why are you so angry? Is that a problem?"
2. "What can we do to help you deal with this?"
3. "I can take the blood pressure for you right now."
4. "Does heart disease or high blood pressure run in your family?"

185. A terminally ill client with multiple myeloma is receiving palliative radiation and increasing doses of morphine sulfate. The client and the nurses have noticed a decline in the physical symptoms of pain. During a care conference, one nurse suggests reducing the morphine and the client's spouse responds, "The people at the hospice said we'll probably never be able to cut back on the pain medicine." The nurse's most therapeutic response would be:
1. "We have to be careful not to cause a physical addiction to narcotics so it's best to reduce the dosage."
2. "The people at the hospice are probably speaking in general terms and are not taking into consideration the uniqueness of this situation."
3. "If we continue increasing the narcotic dose, we may reach the maximum dosage too early. We need to cut back so the drug won't lose its effectiveness."
4. "In many cases, clients with pain from a terminal illness cannot have a reduction in the dosage of pain medicine, but the pain is less now so we can attempt to reduce the dose."

186. The nurse understands that congestive heart failure can best be described as:
    1. An acute state whereby pulmonary circulation pressure decreases
    2. A cardiac condition caused by inadequate circulating blood volume
    3. An inability of the heart to pump blood in proportion to metabolic needs
    4. A chronic state whereby the systolic blood pressure drops below 90 mmHg

187. An 18-year-old client is discharged after having an open reduction and internal fixation of the right femur. The nurse recognizes that discharge teaching was understood when the client states:
    1. "I will have to sit around at home and play video games."
    2. "I will be able to participate in college activities as before."
    3. "There are so many limitations they may as well keep me in the hospital."
    4. "I will be able to move around as long as I elevate my leg every few hours."

188. The nurse teaches the parents of an infant with a cast to evaluate for early signs of decreased circulation from a tight cast. These include:
    1. Swelling or coldness of the toes
    2. Capillary refill of 3 seconds or less
    3. Complaints of numbness or tingling
    4. Blanching of the nail beds with pressure

189. While caring for a neonate receiving phototherapy for physiologic jaundice, the nurse recognizes that this baby is prone to:
    1. Dehydration
    2. Constipation
    3. Respiratory distress
    4. Hypoglycemic reactions

190. Before discharge following a total hip arthroplasty the nurse teaches the client about activity by stating:
    1. "You should climb stairs frequently for exercise."
    2. "You may drive your car after 2 weeks if you desire."
    3. "You should spend most of the day sitting in a comfortable chair."
    4. "You should wear shoes that slip on rather than those with shoe laces."

191. Following a myocardial infarction, a client is in the intensive care unit with an ECG tracing of normal sinus rhythm, which suddenly converts to a rapid dysrhythmia. This dysrhythmia is characterized by extreme irregularity and an absence of atrial activity or QRS complexes. First, the nurse should quickly confirm lead placement on the client and, then:
    1. Prepare for immediate defibrillation
    2. Perform a cardiac thump of the chest
    3. Administer epinephrine IV immediately
    4. Call a code and immediately begin CPR

192. The nursing objective for the child with a congenital heart defect is to keep the child's respiratory rate below 60 breaths per minute. After bathing the child the nurse notes that the respiratory rate is 64. The nurse should:
    1. Update the nursing diagnosis
    2. Notify the physician immediately
    3. Modify the nursing care interventions
    4. Revise the objective to make it more attainable

193. The care plan for a 7-year-old child in traction for a displaced fracture of the femur should have a priority nursing diagnosis of:
    1. Hopelessness related to fear of abandonment
    2. Disturbance in self-esteem related to feelings of shame/guilt
    3. Altered role performance related to change in usual patterns
    4. Diversional activity deficit related to long-term hospitalization

194. The priority nursing diagnosis for a child in the immediate postoperative period following repair of a ventricular septal defect would be:
    1. Impaired gas exchange related to chest pain
    2. High risk for infection related to a thoracic incision
    3. Fluid volume deficit related to nausea and vomiting
    4. Alteration in nutrition related to decreased food intake

195. An HIV positive client visits prenatal services. In response to the client's questions about the transmission of the virus to her fetus, the nurse should base the response on the fact that:
    1. There is a 50% probability the HIV will be transmitted to the fetus during pregnancy
    2. Mother to fetus transmission of HIV can be decreased if the client takes AZT during pregnancy

3. If the pregnant client has not developed AIDS and is merely HIV positive, the fetus will be protected
4. Because of the size of the virus, there is no therapy that can prevent its transmission across the placenta during pregnancy

196. While observing a new mother breastfeeding, the nurse notes that the infant does rhythmic intermittent sucking with the lips spread over the areola and the tongue below the areola. Based on this observation the nurse concludes the baby is:
    1. Positioned properly and nursing effectively
    2. Becoming satisfied and is dropping off to sleep
    3. Nursing ineffectively and will need repositioning
    4. In need of arousal and stimulation to help suck continuously

197. One hour after delivery of a 10 pound 8 ounce baby, a client is found to have a boggy fundus 2 cm above the umbilicus and deviated to the right. The peripad is saturated with bright red lochia and large clots. The nurse palpates a firm round structure above the pubic bone. The nurse's first action should be to:
    1. Assist the woman to empty her bladder
    2. Administer an oxytocic agent as ordered
    3. Massage the uterus until well contracted
    4. Put the baby to breast to stimulate contractions

198. A primigravida at 41 weeks gestation is being admitted to the intrapartum unit for labor induction. To begin planning care the nurse will need to assess for:
    1. Vaginal discharge
    2. Uterine contractions
    3. Status of the membranes
    4. Degree of cervical softness

199. The nurse should suspect that a client has an antisocial personality disorder when the client exhibits:
    1. Empathy, tolerance, intelligence
    2. Mature, future-oriented, generous
    3. Depression, insomnia, remorseful
    4. Charm, impulsiveness, manipulation

200. A 50-year old divorcee, who has lived alone since resigning from an advertising company 5 years ago, enters a mental health diagnostic center because of increasing intellectual impairment. A manifestation of early dementia that the nurse would expect this client to demonstrate would be:
    1. Decreased impulse control
    2. Unpredictable mood changes
    3. A disregard for societal norms
    4. A memory deficit for recent events

201. When assessing a 75-year-old client, the nurse recognizes that a finding not associated with the aging process would be:
    1. A forward-leaning posture
    2. The complaint of ill-fitting dentures
    3. The sunken appearance of the eyes
    4. A short, shuffling gait with no arm swing

202. A 25-year-old married client with ulcerative colitis is scheduled for an ileostomy. The client says, "Well, my sex life is out the window." The most therapeutic response from the nurse would be:
    1. "Let's talk about that."
    2. "It really doesn't have to be that way."
    3. "Your partner will need time to adjust."
    4. "Did you discuss the surgery with your partner?"

203. When taking a health history from the family of a 27-year-old client diagnosed with possible encephalopathy or dementia, the nurse should expect to find a history of:
    1. Lupus erythematosus
    2. Primary hypertension
    3. Insulin-dependent diabetes mellitus
    4. Acquired immunodeficiency syndrome

204. A 75-year-old client with protein malnutrition and obesity undergoes an exploratory laparotomy secondary to severe acute abdominal pain. On the fourth postoperative day after the client ambulates approximately 30 feet and is returned to bed, the nurse notices the large abdominal dressing is saturated with drainage. Before the activity, there was no evidence of wound exudate. The best initial nursing intervention would be for the nurse to:
    1. Splint the abdomen with a pillow and then call the surgeon
    2. Lift the client's dressing gently to directly assess the wound
    3. Brace the client's wound by applying a snug abdominal binder
    4. Reinforce the existing dressing with abdominal combine dressings

205. A client receiving continuous enteral feedings by way of a gastric tube develops nausea and abdominal distention. The nurse assesses the gastric residual, which is 250 mL. The client vomits, develops rapid, labored breathing, and begins losing consciousness. At this point it is most important for the nurse to:
1. Assess the airway and suction it if necessary
2. Decompress the stomach by way of the gastric tube
3. Sit the client up and give supplemental oxygen by mask
4. Position the client supine and prepare for pulmonary resuscitation

206. The nurse reviews the medication schedule with a 12-year-old child who has cystic fibrosis, focusing on when the child is to take the pancreatic enzymes. The statement by the child that would indicate a need for further teaching would be:
1. "I only take enzymes at dinner, when I eat a big meal."
2. "I always take my enzymes right before I eat my food."
3. "When I eat fried foods, I take an extra enzyme capsule."
4. "If I have a snack between meals, I take one enzyme capsule."

207. A risk factor that would necessitate follow-up care for a woman desiring oral contraceptives would be a history of:
1. Endometriosis
2. Breast cancer in the family
3. Pelvic inflammatory disease
4. Hyperthyroidism in the family

208. A client with dementia has been burning food while cooking meals at home. The visiting nurse can be most supportive of this client's attempts at maintaining independence by:
1. Encouraging self-care activities
2. Giving simple one-step directions
3. Suggesting the presence of a relative
4. Arranging for food preparation for the client

209. When assisting a client who is undergoing spousal abuse, it is of primary importance for the nurse to:
1. Identify the client's coping mechanisms
2. Assist the client with anticipatory grieving
3. Urge the client to focus on self-sufficiency

4. Encourage the client to expect feelings of guilt

210. A male client with schizophrenia barricades himself in his room and says, "There are spies everywhere. I need to defend myself." The best nursing response would be:
1. "Spies. Tell me more."
2. "I am your nurse. Let's talk now."
3. "It sounds to me that you are feeling powerful."
4. "You need to come out of your room now, or we will medicate you."

211. The nurse provides active and passive range-of-motion exercises for a 4-year-old child who has had orthopedic surgery for a leg deformity. The client-centered goal related to the range of motion exercises is:
1. Provide recreation and diversion
2. Maintain growth and development
3. Prevent further deformity due to lack of use
4. Avoid injury once ambulation is reestablished

212. During a routine health visit for a 1-year-old child with AIDS, the assessment data that demonstrates normal growth and development would be:
1. Inconsistent eye contact with caretakers
2. Ability to sit alone, but not to crawl or cruise
3. Weight at the 40th percentile on the growth chart
4. Height below the 5th percentile on the growth chart

213. An 85-year-old client fell while jogging and fractured the left hip. Following a total hip replacement, the client is using a walker. The statement by the client that would indicate successful fulfillment of Erikson's eighth developmental task is:
1. "I have been really constipated since I had my surgery because I can't go jogging any more."
2. "You know that I was the engineer who designed the guidance system for the first spacecraft."
3. "The doctor tells me I am doing well with my physical therapy, but I still can't walk by myself."
4. "I may have trouble getting around, but I can continue to paint still life flowers for my grandchildren."

214. An elderly client has been taught to use a walker because of arthritis. The action by the client while using the walker that would indicate the need for further instruction in the proper use of the walker is that the client:
    1. Takes a step then advances the walker
    2. Advances the walker then steps to the walker
    3. Backs walker to a seat when preparing to sit down
    4. Pushes on the arms of a chair to rise to a standing position

215. The nursing intervention that is most therapeutic for a client with arterial blood gases of pH 7.5, PO_2 95 mmHg, PCO_2 30 mmHg, O_2 saturation 95 %, and HCO_2 24 mEq/liter is to:
    1. Administer the prescribed diuretic
    2. Instruct the client to rebreathe exhaled air
    3. Offer the client a favorite carbonated beverage
    4. Administer the prescribed supplemental oxygen

216. A client with a myocardial infarction receives intravenous morphine sulfate to relieve chest pain. A central venous line is to be inserted. Before the procedure, the client's respiratory status was stable. During the procedure, the client develops labored breathing, asymmetrical chest movement, and diminished breath sounds on the side of the insertion site. The nurse would be most accurate in suspecting:
    1. An overdose or hypersensitivity to the morphine sulfate
    2. Possible pneumothorax resulting from the line insertion
    3. Positioning during the procedure is complicating ventilation
    4. The client has had an extension of the myocardial infarction

217. Following a heart transplant, a client is in the cardiothoracic intensive care unit with a Swan-Ganz catheter in place. Eight hours after surgery, the client's blood pressure and central venous pressure (CVP) show a steady decline while the ratio of fluid intake to urine output is increasing. Based on these assessments, it would be most accurate for the nurse to suspect the common postoperative complication of:
    1. Hemorrhage
    2. Heart failure
    3. Dehydration
    4. Transplant rejection

218. A client requires assisted ventilation with the use of positive end expiratory pressure (PEEP). When a ventilator is used:
    1. A tracheostomy must be performed
    2. The client's cardiac output may increase
    3. Oxygen 100% can be given for up to 24 hours
    4. The head must not be raised more than 30 degrees

219. A client has a gastric ulcer that has not responded to antibiotic therapy. After the client undergoes a gastric vagotomy, the nurse would expect an increase in:
    1. Peristalsis
    2. GI motility
    3. The gastric acidity
    4. The pH of gastric juices

220. A female client with severe head injuries is to be placed on a ventilator and intracranial pressure monitoring. The nurse's statement to the client's spouse that would best explain why a ventilator is necessary is:
    1. "Your wife could not breathe on her own and the ventilator is needed to breathe for her."
    2. "Since the oxygen level is low, the ventilator is needed to give your wife additional oxygen."
    3. "The ventilator will help keep your wife's CO_2 low so that swelling in the brain will be decreased."
    4. "Your wife will probably need surgery to relieve pressure on the brain and it is safer to place the ventilator now."

221. A glycosylated hemoglobin assay is ordered for a client with diabetes mellitus. This test is important because it provides information regarding the:
    1. Risk of developing cardiovascular complications
    2. Amount of circulating glycogen available for cell use
    3. Effect of glucose on the production of red blood cells
    4. Blood glucose control over the prior 2-month period

222. A client with schizophrenia, who is receiving haloperidol (Haldol), seems upset and complains of a stiff neck, difficulty swallowing, and tight muscles. The nurse's initial response to these complaints should be to:
1. Assist the client to lie down and relax
2. Stay with the client until calmness returns
3. Administer the prn anticholinergic medication immediately
4. Reassure the client that this is a normal side effect of the medication

223. A client is diagnosed with *Chlamydia trachomatis*. Before prescribing treatment, the nurse practitioner should:
1. Test for gonorrhea
2. Test for diabetes mellitus
3. Determine if the client is pregnant
4. Determine the client's sexual practices

224. On the first postoperative day after a mastectomy, it would be most therapeutic for the client's arm on the affected side to be:
1. Positioned with the arm extended at heart level
2. Placed in a dependent position with pillow support
3. Dressed with an elastic bandage to prevent edema
4. Elevated with the hand and elbow above the shoulder

225. While assessing an antepartal client early in her pregnancy, the nurse observes a slightly enlarged thyroid gland. This is most likely associated with:
1. Iodine deficiency
2. Preexisting thyroid disease
3. An increased metabolic rate
4. An upper respiratory infection

Comprehensive examination 4

226. The nurse, developing a health teaching plan for parents whose child is recovering from bacterial meningitis, should include information on the:
1. Importance of lifelong antibiotic therapy
2. Signs of tuberculosis that should be watched for
3. Actions to be taken if the child develops seizures
4. Need to repeat the dose of *Haemophilus influenzae* type B vaccine

227. A 2-year-old has been diagnosed with conjunctivitis. The nurse's primary goal when caring for this child is to:
1. Keep the eye clean
2. Give oral antibiotics
3. Administer influenza vaccine
4. Provide teaching for parents on vision screening

228. Play is an important aspect of care for a hospitalized child, and the nurse recognizes that to be effective play activities should be:
1. Initiated and controlled by the child
2. Determined by the health care worker
3. Utilized when the parents are not around
4. Explained to the child in order to enhance meaning

229. A client is admitted for surgery for cancer of the bladder. During the admission assessment the nurse would expect the client to complain most often of:
1. Flank pain
2. Urinary stasis
3. Bladder spasms
4. Painless hematuria

230. A couple planning artificial insemination wish to choose the characteristics of the donor. The nurse recommends that they use:
1. A sperm bank
2. In vitro fertilization
3. Donor insemination
4. Husband insemination

231. The nurse recognizes that the client understands post-vasectomy teaching when he states:
1. "I can reverse this surgery at any time."
2. "I know that I am no longer producing sperm."
3. "I will need two follow-up negative sperm counts."

4. "I must avoid sexual intercourse for at least 2 weeks."

232. A client with a mood disorder, manic phase, continually strings words together repeating, "Be, me, gee, he, tea, see." The nurse recognizes this is an example of:
1. Echolalia
2. Word salad
3. Clang association
4. Pressure of speech

233. A middle-aged client has been unable to travel outside of the immediate neighborhood for the past 6 months. The client states, "When I attempt to go downtown, I experience a rapid pulse, and my heart feels like it is pounding out of my chest." The nurse recognizes that the client is reporting a phobic reaction and is using the defense mechanism of:
1. Splitting
2. Projection
3. Repression
4. Displacement

234. Nursing approaches with a client who has a stress related physical illness should focus on the:
1. Effects of the client's illness on the family
2. Meaning of the physical illness to the client
3. Identification of the client's healthy coping mechanisms
4. Relationship between the client's emotions and the physical illness

235. A 68-year-old male client, with a history of prostate problems, is admitted for surgery. A nursing diagnosis with high priority in the postoperative and recovery periods will be:
1. Altered sexual patterns
2. Risk of urinary retention
3. Toileting self-care deficit
4. Risk of fluid volume excess

236. A client who has sustained a basilar fracture of the cranium has rhinorrhea. The nurse tests this drainage for glucose because glucose:
1. Is present in cerebrospinal fluid but not mucus
2. Indicates complications with the pituitary gland
3. Is present in mucus but not in cerebrospinal fluid
4. Indicates increasing cerebral edema and intracranial pressure

52

237. An elderly client, who has recently been widowed, is currently living in an assisted-living care center. The grown children and grandchildren visit regularly. An appropriate long-term goal for meeting this client's developmental needs is:
   1. The client will begin to replace independent role with one of dependency within 2 months
   2. The client will express a sense of ego integrity and psychosocial well-being within 2 months
   3. The client will have cause of social isolation corrected and establish meaningful social contacts within a week
   4. The family will demonstrate support and assistance in fulfilling the client's emotional needs within 2 weeks

238. The nurse observes a client exhibiting nasal flaring, over-use of the trapezius and intercostal muscles, and tripod positioning. These assessments would most support a nursing diagnosis of:
   1. Activity intolerance
   2. Impaired gas exchange
   3. Ineffective airway clearance
   4. Ineffective breathing pattern

239. A client is brought to the emergency department after a motorcycle accident. The client has large abrasions and gaping lacerations on the right side. Before beginning the admission of the client, the nurse should first:
   1. Get gloves and put them on
   2. Assist the client to the Fowler's position
   3. Place an ID band on the client's left wrist
   4. Assess the client for hemorrhage or shock

240. The nurse is aware that the type of schizophrenia that meets the essential criteria of flat or inappropriate affect, incoherent speech, and bizzare behavior is the:
   1. Residual type
   2. Paranoid type
   3. Catatonic type
   4. Disorganized type

241. Outcome criteria for successful treatment of posttraumatic stress syndrome would include a description of the client's ability to:
   1. Sleep through the night
   2. Deal with an altered body image

   3. Verbalize the absence of suicidal thoughts
   4. Describe a feeling of control over ritualistic behaviors

242. Therapeutic management of a child with rheumatic fever should focus on:
   1. Preventing chorea
   2. Bedrest during the acute phase
   3. Compliance with steroid therapy
   4. Placing the child in respiratory isolation

243. The nurse teaches the parents of a newborn infant that they should call for medical advice if vomiting and/or diarrhea are present and:
   1. Persist for 3 days
   2. Continue over an 8-hour period
   3. The infant vomits once and has one watery stool
   4. Voiding is occurring about once every 2 to 3 hours

244. A woman who is pregnant has preexisting cystic fibrosis. In relation to her diet, the nurse should instruct the client to:
   1. Decrease proteins
   2. Increase iron intake
   3. Increase carbohydrates
   4. Decrease calcium intake

245. The nurse plans to notify the pediatrician when, during the newborn assessment, the nurse observes:
   1. A negative tonic-neck reflex
   2. The harlequin sign when sleeping
   3. A positive Babinski reflex on both feet
   4. The ears below the outer canthus of the eyes

246. When symptoms of weight gain, oily skin, hirsutism, and atrophic vaginitis occur, the action by the nurse that would be most appropriate for the client who is using danozol (Danocrine) for endometriosis is to:
   1. Suggest that the client consider becoming pregnant
   2. Speak to the physician about discontinuing the drug
   3. Schedule surgical intervention as ordered by the physician
   4. Recommend that the client consider hormone replacement therapy

247. When a nurse administers antipsychotic medications to clients in psychiatric units, the theoretical model being used to provide a framework for understanding client behaviors is:
1. Biologic
2. Systems
3. Cognitive
4. Psychoanalytic

248. When caring for a client who is experiencing delirium tremens, it is important for the nurse to:
1. Promote sleep through the use of sedatives
2. Keep the room dimly lit to promote relaxation
3. Closely monitor vital signs to evaluate progress
4. Ensure client safety through the use of restraints

249. A community-based anticipatory guidance activity that could provide skills to prevent a maturational crisis would be:
1. A fire prevention program
2. Rape-crisis intervention service
3. Pre-retirement counseling program
4. Formulation of a community disaster plan

250. The initial nursing approach for interrupting hallucinatory behavior in clients should focus on:
1. Establishing rapport with the client
2. Assuring that the client has an order for antipsychotic medication
3. Teaching the client about activities that can be used to distract from the hallucinations
4. Exploring the possible reasons for the increase in anxiety the client is probably experiencing

251. The most sensitive measurement of renal function is:
1. Specific gravity
2. Serum creatinine
3. Renal ultrasonography
4. BUN (Blood urea nitrogen)

252. Shortly after admission a client, who has sustained a blunt frontal head injury, has a generalized tonic clonic seizure. The most important nursing intervention during the tonic clonic phase is to:
1. Establish a patent airway
2. Protect the client from self-injury
3. Closely monitor the client's vital signs
4. Record the sequence of the seizure activity

253. Intravenous phenytoin (Dilantin) 500 mg is being administered to a client. The nurse understands that the drug must be infused slowly because:
1. Severe hypotension and vascular collapse can occur
2. Status epilepticus results if the infusion is too rapid
3. Venous toxicity occurs when IV phenytoin is administered rapidly
4. Drowsiness and confusion may occur and mask signs of increased intracranial pressure

254. A client who has had a transurethral resection of the prostate (TURP) has had the catheter removed. The nurse can best meet the needs of this client at risk for urinary retention by:
1. Catheterizing the client whenever voiding has not occurred in 8 hours
2. Assisting the client to attempt voiding at regular intervals to prevent distention if possible
3. Giving the client ordered pain medication at regular intervals to decrease any discomfort with voiding or during catheterization
4. Allowing the bladder to fill and be palpable before attempting to assist in voiding since a fully distended bladder produces more stimulation to void

255. When teaching the parents of a child with sickle cell anemia the importance of promoting adequate oxygenation it would be important for the nurse to:
1. Suggest relocation to a higher altitude
2. Explain how demand is altered by infection
3. Recommend daily damp dusting and mopping
4. Encourage a dietary intake of fruits and vegetables

256. The nurse explains to the parents of a child with anemia that the most accurate statement about the problem with the blood is that the:
1. Viscosity of the blood is increased
2. Shape of the erythrocytes is altered
3. Hematopoietic system is depressed
4. Oxygen-carrying capacity of the blood is decreased

257. Nursing intervention to aid the trauma victim's family should be considered effective if the family:

1. Maintains a familiar pattern of functioning
2. Directs anger or guilt away from the event
3. Avoids emotion-focused coping responses
4. Achieves a realistic perception of the event

258. Prior to interviewing the parents of a child who has been sexually abused, the nurse should be:
1. Familiar with personal feelings about sexual abuse
2. Cognizant of the legal ramifications of sexual abuse
3. Aware of the fact that abusing families are highly dysfunctional
4. Knowledgeable of community resources available for the child and the family

259. A nurse is assigned to establish a one-to-one relationship with a young schizophrenic client. The nurse could best gain the client's consent and agreement by stating:
1. "I will interview you each day for 9 weeks."
2. "I would like to talk with you regularly about your problem."
3. "I want to meet with you at 9 AM each morning in your room."
4. "I would like to meet with you every day and give you the opportunity to talk about things that are of concern to you."

260. When the nurse cares for a client with diabetes mellitus, it is essential to be aware that other physiologic conditions or therapy can affect insulin demand or response. Safe, comprehensive care requires the nurse to recognize that:
1. The pregnant client with diabetes mellitus may have a reduced insulin requirement
2. Clients taking beta blockers may not experience the usual early signals of low blood glucose
3. Cigarette smoking speeds insulin absorption if the client smokes within 30 minutes of the injection
4. Starting or stopping an exercise program will not affect insulin need as long as the diet remains unchanged

261. A client with a head injury develops an excessive increase in urine output with a urine specific gravity of 1.001. The change in the client's condition is reported to the physician. The medication that the nurse would expect the physician to order is:
1. Insulin
2. Dilantin

3. Decadron
4. Vasopressin

262. After reviewing the laboratory tests of a client who has had an abruptio placentae, the nurse notes a normal CBC with an increased prothrombin time and a decreased fibrinogen and platelet count. The nurse suspects:
1. Hemophilia
2. Hypofibrinogenemia
3. Postpartum hemorrhage
4. Disseminated intravascular coagulopathy

263. A client in active labor is to have an epidural block. While this is being administered, the nursing action that takes priority is:
1. Checking the uterine contractions for an increase in strength
2. Positioning the mother flat in bed to avoid postspinal headache
3. Telling the mother she will feel the need to void more frequently
4. Monitoring the maternal blood pressure for possible hypotension

264. During mastectomy surgery, a negative pressure drainage apparatus is inserted to drain the client's surgical site. Eight hours postoperatively, the drain's collection chamber contains 200 mL of blood. Interpretation of this finding should lead the nurse to:
1. Filter and then reinfuse the drainage
2. Drain the chamber and recharge the drain
3. Clamp the drain tubing and notify the physician
4. Assess the client for signs of excessive blood loss

265. When assessing a child with tetralogy of Fallot, the nurse observes that the fingers and toes are:
1. Pallid and tapered
2. Purplish and clubbed
3. Reddened and stubby
4. Blanched and elongated

266. The nurse recognizes that postoperative education for a 5-year-old following an appendectomy has been successful when the child can:
1. Ask a parent to request an analgesic
2. Utilize a pain rating scale appropriately
3. Verbalize the type and amount of pain present
4. Request analgesia when pain becomes distressful

267. The nurse is aware that an essential feature of the dementia found in clients with a history of repeated head injuries, such as boxers, is usually:
1. Somewhat transitory
2. Progressive in nature
3. Limited to motor or sensory deficits
4. Associated with postural instability and resting tremors

268. During the termination phase of a nurse-client relationship, the statement that indicates the client is beginning to experience separation anxiety would be:
1. "We had a party here last night. It was fun."
2. "I have made a decision to go back to my job."
3. "I have enjoyed these meetings and our relationship."
4. "I was thinking about what I will do when I leave here."

269. A client with a 2-month history of urinary frequency and a 20-year history of diabetes mellitus is scheduled for a cystoscopy at 10 AM after being NPO since the night before. At 6:30 on the morning of the procedure, a nurse collects a capillary blood sample and using a capillary blood glucose monitor finds the capillary blood glucose to be 45 mg/dL. The client is alert, clearly verbal, and denies hypoglycemic symptoms. The nurse's initial response should be to:
1. Give the client orange juice and sugar
2. Start Dextrose 50 g IV infusion immediately
3. Assess the capillary blood glucose a second time
4. Document the finding and withhold the morning insulin

270. The nurse is aware that a 72-year-old female with ill-fitting dentures needs further nutritional instruction when the client states:
1. "I can't find many cereals that have both raisins and nuts in them."
2. "I made liver and onions last week, but my husband did not like it."
3. "I have been eating a lot of spinach and now my bowel movements are really dark."
4. "My husband and I have decided the bean and pea soups I started making are really great."

271. Four months ago, an adult client experienced a complete transection injury at the fourth (4th) lumbar vertebra. The nurse plans a client education program in anticipation of the client's discharge 1 week from now. The nurse would assign the highest priority to teaching strategies for:
1. Managing dysreflexic episodes
2. Transferring in and out of automobiles
3. Creating alternatives for sexual expression
4. Maintaining bowel and bladder elimination

272. A client with a long-standing history of end stage renal disease (ESRD) is admitted for diagnostic studies of cardiovascular status. The nurse plans the client's schedule in anticipation of the client's:
1. Risk for fluid volume deficit
2. Probable activity intolerance
3. Increased risk for hemorrhage
4. Desire to actively participate in decision-making

273. An active 80-year-old has sustained a hip fracture and has had a hip replacement. The client is currently using a walker. The goal that would be most important in providing for the client's safety needs at discharge is:
1. Promote maximum degree of independent self-care
2. Prevent any complications secondary to the immobility
3. Arrange for acceptable living arrangements post discharge
4. Compensate for sensory deficits through the use of assistive devices

274. A client who has had a colostomy asks how to prevent odors. The nurse's best response would be:
1. "Eating cucumbers, asparagus, turnips, and peas will help prevent odor."
2. "AquaMEPHYTON will decrease the decompostion of blood and prevent odor."
3. "The Nystatin swish and swallow the physician ordered will decrease odor-causing bacteria."
4. "Dark green vegetables, especially parsley, and more vitamin C in the diet will help the odor problem."

275. A full-term infant is now 2 days old and is being breastfed. The nurse notes that the skin appears somewhat yellow and suspects that the infant is experiencing:
1. Indirect jaundice
2. Asphytic jaundice
3. Pathologic jaundice
4. Physiologic jaundice

276. The nurse in the newborn nursery has just been informed that a newly admitted baby boy has hypospadius. The nurse expects the examination of his genitalia to reveal:
1. That one or both of his testes have not descended into the scrotal sac
2. The urethral opening above the glans penis along the dorsal surface of the penile shaft
3. A palpable bulge in the inguinal or scrotal area as a result of fluid in the persistent processus vaginalis
4. The urethral opening just below the glans penis or anywhere along the ventral surface of the penile shaft

277. A 5-year-old in bilateral femoral skeletal traction is found by the nurse with the 5-pound weights resting on the floor. The nurse's priority intervention would be to:
1. Position the child so the weights hang free
2. Note whether the traction is in the proper position
3. Notify the physician to decrease the traction cord lengths
4. Remove a weight from each leg until the weights hang free

278. A 10-year-old with cystic fibrosis is receiving dornase alpha (DNase, Pulmozyme) therapy. The nurse should plan to initiate chest physiotherapy:
1. Before meals
2. Before each DNase dose
3. When the child requests it
4. After each IV antibiotic dose

279. When caring for a client with dementia who is exhibiting agitation, it would be most therapeutic for the nurse to:
1. Scold the client for the acting-out behavior
2. Turn on the TV in the client's room as a distraction
3. Apply restraints, then leave the client to quiet down
4. Explore the possible meaning of the behavior to the client

280. A client with diabetes mellitus develops peripheral arterial disease and complains of pain in the lower extremities. The nurse should teach the client to:
1. Apply heat to promote blood flow
2. Maintain rest to decrease O_2 needs
3. Wear snug shoes to discourage swelling
4. Avoid smoking to prevent vasoconstriction

281. A client whose blood pressure has been increasing throughout her pregnancy calls the prenatal clinic at 36 weeks gestation complaining of a dull headache, some confusion, and severe heartburn. The nurse's best response would be:
1. "Tell me everything you ate yesterday and today."
2. "Please stay on the line. I'm calling an ambulance for you."
3. "Please drive to the clinic immediately. Do you think you can make it?"
4. "Take some enteric-coated Tylenol and Maalox. If that does not help, please call back."

282. Immediately after delivery a client begins to shake uncontrollably. The best nursing intervention at this time would be to:
1. Take the client's temperature
2. Cover the client with a warm blanket
3. Notify the client's physician immediately
4. Encourage the client to take slow, deep breaths

283. A primigravida in early labor tells the nurse that she has back pain. The most appropriate activity for the nurse to suggest would be to:
1. Rock and tilt the pelvis
2. Perform the Kegel exercise
3. Elevate the legs above the hips
4. Breathe by pretending to blow out a candle

284. A client is receiving total parenteral nutrition (TPN). A significant change in vital signs that would require the nurse to take action is:
1. Pulse rate of 76 changing to 64
2. BP of 140/90 changing to 112/82
3. Temperature of 97° changing to 99.4°
4. Respiratory rate of 16 changing to 22

285. The nurse has provided discharge teaching to a client who has had a total laryngectomy. The nurse evaluates that the teaching is understood when the client writes:
1. "It isn't necessary for me to quit smoking."
2. "I won't be able to go swimming anymore."
3. "I won't need to make any life-style changes."
4. "There's no need to cover the stoma when I go out."

286. Following a liver biopsy the nurse checks a client's dressing and notices a moderately large amount of bile-colored drainage. The client also complains of right upper quadrant pain. The nurse should recognize that:
1. The pancreas has been lacerated
2. A biliary vessel has been penetrated
3. This is the normal, expected response
4. Fluid is probably leaking into the intestine

287. The nurse would expect blood values in a 5-year-old with status asthmaticus to indicate:
1. A pH of 7.32, a PCO_2 of 60 mmHg, and a PO_2 of 70 mmHg
2. A pH of 7.35, a PCO_2 of 45 mmHg, and a PO_2 of 88 mmHg
3. A pH of 7.46, a PCO_2 of 30 mmHg, and a PO_2 of 90 mmHg
4. A pH of 7.40, a PCO_2 of 40 mmHg, and a PO_2 of 80 mmHg

288. The nurse evaluates the effectiveness of respiratory care for an adolescent with cystic fibrosis by:
1. Taking sputum cultures
2. Sending the client to the bicycling room
3. Monitoring vital signs and pulse oxymetry values
4. Assessing frequency of requests for chest physiotherapy

289. A client has been diagnosed as having cancer of the lung. When performing a history and physical the nurse should assess for:
1. Dysphagia
2. Hemoptysis
3. Hoarseness
4. Lymphadenopathy

290. The nurse is aware that a physiologic change of aging that can affect surgical outcomes is:
1. Increased cardiac output
2. Decreased glucocorticoid secretion
3. Decreased glomerular filtration rate
4. Increased elasticity of pulmonary tissue

291. A client with pneumothorax has a chest tube inserted. The tube is attached to an underwater drainage system with 20 cm of suction. At 3:00 PM, 300 mL of yellowish drainage and continuous fluctuations in the water-seal chamber are reported. At 5:00 PM, the drainage has streaks of blood and is at the 500 mL level. The nurse should:

1. Milk the chest tube to prevent it from clogging
2. Assess the client's respiratory status every hour
3. Notify the physician and assess the client more frequently
4. Check the client's blood pressure and the chest tube drainage every 4 hours

292. A client just diagnosed with insulin-dependent diabetes mellitus is admitted to the hospital with diabetic ketoacidosis. The nurse would expect to note:
1. Hunger and fatigue
2. Palpitations and anxiety
3. Diaphoresis and confusion
4. Rapid breathing and dehydration

293. The nursing intervention that would best assist in meeting the needs of a client with lung cancer is:
1. Placing in the semi-Fowler's position and administering supplemental humidified oxygen
2. Providing a morphine drip to alleviate pain and placing in high-Fowler's position to promote airway expansion
3. Administering prescribed analgesic for the pain radiating back to the flank that limits deep breathing and providing postural drainage
4. Supporting use of accessory chest muscles while providing supplemental oxygen via tent and bronchoconstrictors to decrease inflammation

294. A client with bladder cancer, who had both radiation and an ileal conduit, is tested for the presence of carcinoembryonic antigen (CEA). The client asks the nurse what decreased amounts of this protein mean. The best reply by the nurse would be:
1. This protein needs to be replaced since it is needed for normal cell metabolism
2. The immune system was overwhelmed and the tumor growth may be out of control
3. The ability to develop antibodies (cellular immunity) to fight the tumor growth is diminished
4. The decrease in this tumor-associated antigen probably reflects successful therapy and tumor regression

295. The nurse assesses that a client who has had a total laryngectomy is ready to begin oral feedings when the client:

58

1. Can whisper softly
2. Is 24 hours post surgery
3. Begins to swallow saliva
4. Has a return of peristalsis

296. The nurse has completed teaching self-care to an adult with insulin-dependent diabetes mellitus. The nurse determines teaching has been effective when the client states:
    1. "You can count on me; I do what I'm told. I'm going to be real good so I won't have any problems."
    2. "Now that I know about the diabetes, I need to stay close to my doctor and keep my diet within a regular schedule."
    3. "If someday I have dessert or eat a bit more than usual, I can take a little extra insulin so the sugar doesn't get too high."
    4. "I should check my blood sugar level four times a day and record it on this log, and take the log when I go to the doctor."

297. A 3-month-old is brought into the emergency department at 4:00 AM and could not be resuscitated. The teenage mother found the baby not breathing, ashen in color and cold, with a blanket clutched to the baby's face. Crying hysterically, the mother states, "My baby was fine, with just a slight cold." The nurse recognizes that the diagnosis probably will be:
    1. Apnea of infancy
    2. Bronchopulmonary dysplasia
    3. Sudden infant death syndrome
    4. Respiratory distress syndrome

298. The finding in the newborn that indicates a need for further assessment is:
    1. A positive Babinski reflex
    2. Overriding sagittal sutures
    3. An umbilical cord with two vessels
    4. Three-second pauses in respirations

299. The individual who has the highest risk of developing breast cancer is a woman who is:
    1. Nulliparous, had an early menarche, and a late menopause
    2. Thirty years old, had an oophorectomy, and consumes a low-fat diet
    3. Thirty-five years old, had a late menarche, and an early menopause
    4. Multiparous, had an early first pregnancy, and consumes a high-fat diet

300. The nursing care plan for a pregnant client being treated for preterm labor should include:
    1. Diet to counteract protein loss from inactivity
    2. Activities to counteract boredom from bed rest
    3. Fluid restriction to decrease trips to the bathroom
    4. Assessment for side effects of oxytocic medications

Appendix A
State and Territorial Boards of Nursing

Alabama

Board of Nursing
RSA Plaza, Suite 250
770 Washington Avenue
Montgomery, Alabama 36130

Alaska

Board of Nursing
Department of Commerce & Economic Development
Division of Occupational Licensing
P.O. Box 110806
Juneau, Alaska 99811-0806

Arizona

Board of Nursing
1651 East Morten, Suite 150
Phoenix, Arizona 85020

Arkansas

Board of Nursing
University Tower Building, Suite 800
1123 S. University Avenue
Little Rock, Arkansas 72204

California

Board of Registered Nursing
P.O. Box 944210
400 R Street, Suite 4030
Sacramento, California 95814-6200

Colorado

Board of Nursing
1560 Broadway, Suite 670
Denver, Colorado 80202

Connecticut

Board of Examiners for Nursing
150 Washington Street
Hartford, Connecticut 06106

Delaware

Board of Nursing
Cannon Building
P.O. Box 1401
861 Silver Lake Boulevard
Dover, Delaware 19903-1401

District of Columbia

Board of Nursing
614 H. Street NW
Washington, D.C. 20001

Florida

Board of Nursing
111 E. Coastline Drive, Suite 516
Jacksonville, Florida 32202

Georgia

Board of Nursing
166 Pryor Street SW, Suite 400
Atlanta, Georgia 30303

Guam

Board of Nurse Examiners
Box 2816
Agana, Guam 96910

Hawaii

Board of Nursing
Box 3469
Honolulu, Hawaii 96801

Idaho

Board of Nursing
P.O. Box 83720
2800 N. 8th Street, Suite 210
Boise, Idaho 83720-0061

Illinois

Department of Professional Regulation
320 W. Washington Street, 3rd Floor
Springfield, Illinois 62786

Indiana

State Board of Nursing
Health Professions Bureau
402 W. Washington Street, Room 041
Indianapolis, Indiana 46204

Iowa

Board of Nursing
1223 E. Court
Des Moines, Iowa 50319

Kansas

State Board of Nursing
Landon State Office Bldg.
900 SW Jackson, Room 551-S
Topeka, Kansas 66612-1230

Kentucky

Board of Nursing
312 Whittington Parkway, Suite 300
Louisville, Kentucky 40222-5172

Louisiana

Board of Nursing
150 Baronne Street, Room 912
New Orleans, Louisiana 70112

Maine

Board of Nursing
35 Anthony Avenue
State House Station 158
Augusta, Maine 04333

Maryland

Board of Nursing
4140 Patterson Avenue
Baltimore, Maryland 21215-2254

Massachusetts

Board of Registration in Nursing
Government Center
100 Cambridge Street, Room 1519
Boston, Massachusetts 02202

Michigan

Board of Nursing
P.O. Box 30018
Lansing, Michigan 48909

Minnesota

Board of Nursing
2700 University Avenue W, Suite 108
St. Paul, Minnesota 55114

Mississippi

Board of Nursing
239 N. Lamar Street, Suite 401
Jackson, Mississippi 39201

Missouri

Board of Nursing
3605 Missouri Blvd.
P.O. Box 656
Jefferson City, Missouri 65102

Montana

Board of Nursing
Department of Commerce
P.O. Box 200513
111 N. Jackson
Helena, Montana 59620-0513

Nebraska

Board of Nursing
P.O. Box 95007
Lincoln, Nebraska 68509

Nevada

Board of Nursing
1281 Terminal Way, Suite 116
Reno, Nevada 89502

New Hampshire

Board of Nursing
Division of Public Health Services
Health & Welfare Building
6 Hazen Drive
Concord, New Hampshire 03301

New Jersey

Board of Nursing
124 Halsey Street
Newark, New Jersey 07102

New Mexico

Board of Nursing
4206 Louisiana Boulevard NE
Albuquerque, New Mexico 87109-1807

New York

Board of Nursing
New York State Education Department, Room 3023
Cultural Education Center
Albany, New York 12230

North Carolina

Board of Nursing
P.O. Box 2129
Raleigh, North Carolina 27602-2129

North Dakota

Board of Nursing
919 S. 7th Street, Suite 504
Bismarck, North Dakota 58504-5881

Ohio

Board of Nursing
77 S. High Street, 17th Floor
Columbus, Ohio 43266-0316

Oklahoma

Board of Nursing
2915 N. Classen Boulevard, Suite 524
Oklahoma City, Oklahoma 73106

Oregon

Board of Nursing
800 NE Oregon Street, Suite 465
Portland, Oregon 97232

Pennsylvania

Board of Nursing
P.O. Box 2649
Harrisburg, Pennsylvania 17105-2649

Puerto Rico

Board of Nurse Examiners
Call Box 10200
Santurce, Puerto Rico 00908-0200

Rhode Island

Board of Nursing Registration and Education
Cannon Health Building, Room 104
3 Capitol Hill
Providence, Rhode Island 02908-5097

South Carolina

Board of Nursing
Winthrop Building
220 Executive Center Drive, Suite 220
Columbia, South Carolina 29210-8422

South Dakota

Board of Nursing
3307 S. Lincoln Avenue
Sioux Falls, South Dakota 57105

Tennessee

Board of Nursing
Bureau of Manpower and Facilities
283 Plus Park Boulevard
Nashville, Tennessee 37247-1010

Texas

Board of Nurse Examiners
9101 Burnet Road, Suite 104
Austin, Texas 78758

Utah

Board of Nursing
Heber M. Wells Building, 4th Floor
160 E. 300 South
PO Box 45805
Salt Lake City, Utah 84145-0805

Vermont

Board of Nursing
109 State Street
Montpelier, Vermont 05609-1106

Virgin Islands

Board of Nurse Licensure
Kongens Gade #3
P.O. Box 4247
St. Thomas, Virgin Islands 00803

Virginia

Board of Nursing
6606 West Broad Street, 4th Floor
Richmond, Virginia 23230

Washington

Washington State Nursing Care
Quality Assurance Commission
P.O. Box 47864
Olympia, Washington 98504-7864

West Virginia

Board of Examiners for RNs
101 Dee Drive
Charleston, West Virginia 25311

Wisconsin

Board of Nursing
1400 E. Washington Avenue, Room 174
P.O. Box 8935
Madison, Wisconsin 53708-8935

Wyoming

Board of Nursing
Barrett Bldg., 2nd Floor
2301 Central Avenue
Cheyenne, Wyoming 82002

Appendix B
Canadian Provincial Registered Nurses Associations

Alberta

Alberta Association of Registered Nurses
11620 168th Street
Edmonton, Alberta
T5M 4A6
(403) 451-0043

British Columbia

Registered Nurses Association of British Columbia
2855 Arbutus Street
Vancouver, British Columbia
V6Y 3Y8
(604) 736-7731

Manitoba

Manitoba Association of Registered Nurses
647 Broadway Avenue
Winnipeg, Manitoba
R3C 0X2
(204) 774-3477

New Brunswick

Nurses Association of New Brunswick
231 Saunders Street
Fredericton, New Brunswick
E3B 1N6
(506) 458-8731

Newfoundland

Association of Registered Nurses of Newfoundland
55 Military Road
P.O. Box 6116
St. John's, Newfoundland
A1C 5X8
(709) 753-6040

Northwest Territories

Northwest Territories Registered Nurses Association
P.O. Box 2757
Yellowknife, Northwest Territories
X1A 2R1
(403) 873-2745

Nova Scotia

Registered Nurses Association of Nova Scotia
6035 Coburg Road
Halifax, Nova Scotia
B3H 1Y8
(902) 423-6156

Ontario

College of Nurses of Ontario
101 Davenport Road
Toronto, Ontario
M5R 3PI
(416) 928-0900

Prince Edward Island

Association of Nurses of Prince Edward Island
PO Box 1838
Charlottetown, Prince Edward Island
C1A 7N5
(902) 892-6322

Quebec

Ordre des infirmières et infirmiers du Quebec
4200 Quest, Boulevard Dorchester
Montreal, Quebec
H3Z 1V4
(514) 935-2501

Saskatchewan

Saskatchewan Registered Nurses Association
2066 Retallack Street
Regina, Saskatchewan
S4T 2K2
(306) 757-4643

Yukon

Yukon Nurses Society
P.O. Box 5371
Whitehorse, Yukon
Y1A 4Z2
(403) 667-4062